To the Fullest

LORRAINE BRACCO

AND LISA V. DAVIS
WITH DIANE REVERAND

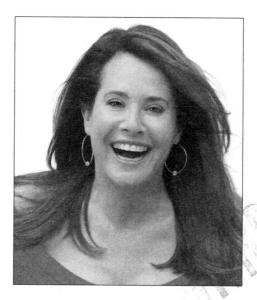

To the Fullest

The Clean Up Your Act Plan to Lose Weight, Rejuvenate, and Be the Best You Can Be

RODALE.

This book is intended as a reference volume only, not as a medical manual. The information given here is designed to help you make informed decisions about your health. It is not intended as a substitute for any treatment that may have been prescribed by your doctor. If you suspect that you have a medical problem, we urge you to seek competent medical help.

The information in this book is meant to supplement, not replace, proper exercise training. All forms of exercise pose some inherent risks. The editors and publisher advise readers to take full responsibility for their safety and know their limits. Before practicing the exercises in this book, be sure that your equipment is well-maintained, and do not take risks beyond your level of experience, aptitude, training, and fitness. The exercise and dietary programs in this book are not intended as a substitute for any exercise routine or dietary regimen that may have been prescribed by your doctor. As with all exercise and dietary programs, you should get your doctor's approval before beginning.

Mention of specific companies, organizations, or authorities in this book does not imply endorsement by the author or publisher, nor does mention of specific companies, organizations, or authorities imply that they endorse this book, its author, or the publisher.

Internet addresses and telephone numbers given in this book were accurate at the time it went to press.

The cleanse discussed by the authors includes some products in which they have a financial gain.

Rodale books may be purchased for business or promotional use or for special sales. For information, please write to: Special Markets Department, Rodale Inc., 733 Third Avenue, New York, NY 10017.

Printed in the United States of America

Rodale Inc. makes every effort to use acid-free ⊗, recycled paper ♻.

The Dirty Dozen and Clean Fifteen Plus lists on page 135 are copyrighted by the Environmental Working Group, www.ewg.org. Reprinted with permission.

The lists of mercury content in fish on pages 137–138 are reprinted with permission from the Natural Resources Defense Council.

The illustration on page 74 is from iStock.

Book design by Amy C. King
Illustrations by MCKIBILLO

Library of Congress Cataloging-in-Publication Data is on file with the publisher.
ISBN-13: 978-1-62336-492-2 hardcover

Distributed to the trade by Macmillan
2 4 6 8 10 9 7 5 3 1 hardcover

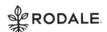

We inspire and enable people to improve their lives and the world around them.
rodalebooks.com

For my parents, who woke me up . . .

When people undermine your dreams, predict your doom, or criticize you, remember they're telling you their story, not yours.

—Cynthia Occelli

If you want something you've never had, then you've got to do something you've never done.

—Attributed to Thomas Jefferson

Without leaps of imagination, or dreaming, we lose the excitement of possibilities. Dreaming, after all, is a form of planning.

—Gloria Steinem

I choose to live by choice, not by chance; to make changes, not excuses; to be motivated and not manipulated; to be useful, not used; to excel, not compete. I choose self-esteem, not self-pity. I choose to listen to my inner voice, not the random opinions of others.

—Author Unknown

CONTENTS

FOREWORD

It is with great pleasure that I have the opportunity to help spread the word to get more people healthy in a way they may not have thought possible. All too often we lose sight of what good health really is. We grow accustomed to not feeling well. In fact, we forget what feeling well is like anymore.

Many of us simply attribute that to age. That is a big cop-out, if you ask me. There is a way to age younger. In my practice, I use the term *immunosenescence*—in other words, immunity rot—to describe the way people start to feel because of the damage they inflict upon themselves each day.

Once you can identify the root cause of a problem, you can get your life back again and feel better than you have in years. Imagine having the energy of your 20-year-old self, not catching the cold that is going around, sleeping solidly, not feeling creaky in the mornings, and jumping out of bed ready to seize each and every day.

It's possible, and *To the Fullest* is a wonderful way to begin your journey back to health. Although Ms. Bracco may be more famous than you and I, you are absolutely going to be able to identify with her struggles and that sensation of "how did I get here?" along with "how do I get out of here?"

I can't tell you how many patients I see who describe a sense of powerlessness on the road to not feeling well. It slowly creeps up on you—every decade, there's another 10 pounds. Every decade, there's another health issue or two that we attribute to getting older. And then, when you think you've finally reached rock bottom, you know it's time to clean up your act.

So, where do you turn? *To the Fullest* is a great place to start. The program outlined in this book is not your ordinary, run-of-the-mill cleanse from the local health food store. It is a clinically tested, well-researched, grounded-in-science system designed to get your body functioning the way it is supposed to function. And not only that, the only side effect is . . . weight loss. Yes, you can use this system if you just want to lose weight, but the program in this book will help you get your life and your health back. It's designed to rejuvenate you so that you can be the best *you* that you can be.

Lorraine does a wonderful job of explaining exactly how this detoxification process works. The scientific material about the cleanse and why she eliminated certain foods from her diet is powerful. I am sure you know friends, family members, or acquaintances who are doing or have done a "detox" or a "cleanse." This is not one of those. This cleanse will seriously make you feel better and not just temporarily. This program will change your life.

Our bodies are fascinating machines that were never meant to handle the overwhelming amount of processed foods, genetically engineered foods, and sugar that the average American eats every single day without even thinking twice about it. The food manufacturers have the marketing machine very well oiled. They have managed to pull the wool over our eyes so effectively that we no longer have the ability to distinguish what is healthy from what is not.

And believe me, there is a lot of money to be made in this burgeoning obesity epidemic. With obesity comes many illnesses. If people eat more, guess who gets rich? The food manufacturers, the big pharmaceutical companies, and, I'm sure, countless politicians who allow this to happen to you, the American public. There is no doubt in my mind as to why we get sick and why so many people suffer needlessly. When I met Lorraine, it was kismet. Our brains, our thought processes, and practically our synapses were in line with how to get America healthy again.

I see many patients in my practice who are just like Lorraine. Starting with a detox protocol is their first step on the road to health improvement. The liver is the organ that clears almost everything. It gets rid of all the toxins, stores energy, and produces cholesterol. This hardworking organ is assaulted every day, practically hourly, because of our toxic lifestyles. That's why it is so important to cleanse this overburdened organ periodically. Could you imagine not cleaning the filter in your air conditioner, dryer, or anything else with a filter? Of course, you wouldn't. The same holds true for your liver, which is the most important filter you will ever have to clean.

You don't have to take my word for this or even Lorraine's word. We each performed our own informal clinical trial. Granted, neither trial was done as rigorously as if we were introducing a new drug, but each one was a good first step that confirmed for both of us—not that we needed convincing—that a good liver detox is a great place to start to improve your health.

Rodale, the publisher of this book, and Lorraine recruited 14 women and one man who wanted to feel better. By the end of the 6-week trial, each one of them had accomplished that and had also lost weight. They couldn't believe how easy it had been. When you read the program and see that you aren't allowed to eat the first 2 days, you are going to think that's impossible. Let me tell you, it isn't. The testimonials you will find scattered throughout the book attest to the fact that it's not that hard.

In the small trial of 10 patients that I performed in my office, not one person complained about hunger during those 2 days. Two mentioned that they were a little tired, which I explained was par for the course with any detoxification, but they were all amazed at the energy level they eventually felt. One of my participants, in fact, had not been able to lose weight or feel better in 10 years, and she was only 33. She had been told she had fibromyalgia and was on multiple medications, and she couldn't lose weight even if she starved herself.

Today, that girl continues to lose weight and has the energy she had when she was in her twenties. We have begun to reduce her medications. She is thrilled, and so am I. I should also mention that all 10 of my patients felt better and more energized, and had an average weight loss of 6 pounds in the first month that they followed the program—and one of them was a man.

Men aren't used to having to suffer for their health. Many of them take a very laissez-faire attitude. Usually something dramatic has to happen, such as a heart attack, before they are frightened enough to do something for themselves. And they are afraid. Women make most of the health decisions in this country anyway, so I am telling all the women who buy this book to do this program as a couple. Why not both start out with fresh, new, healthier bodies?

There is only one way to rid yourself of the stored accumulated toxins, and that is with a liver detox shake and nutritional supplements. But, as I tell my patients, the key element to health and the key element to feeling better is eating in a more healthful manner. This is not a craze or the newest fad protocol. I have been a proponent of what Lorraine says in this book for my entire medical career. The bottom line is that sugar kills. If it were up to me, there would be warning labels on candy bars and soda cans. Simple carbohydrates and any other disguised sugar are also the enemy. Lorraine exposes in full detail the hidden sugars that marketers don't want you to know about. No matter what diet or which diet doctor you believe, there isn't a one of us who feels that sugar is good for you—it isn't your friend. It's time to say your good-byes.

As for processed foods, genetically engineered foods, dairy, foods with antibiotics and growth hormones, animals fed foods that they shouldn't be eating in the first place—these all make us sick and toxic. If you think all the attention on gluten is just the latest fad, it's not and here's why: The wheat we eat in this country is a genetically modified product that doesn't even resemble the wheat our ancestors ate on a molecular level. I'm not referring to ancient ancestors, I mean a mere 50 years ago.

People are getting sick from the foods they eat because the technology has changed so dramatically and quickly in the last 50 years—more than ever before in history. Our bodies are genetically very slow to adapt. We are suffering the consequences with our health and well-being. *To the Fullest* will provide you with the tools to rid your body of a life's worth of toxins and educate you on how to live with minimal exposure to these harmful substances forever. This is the jump start we all could use.

Though I practice and preach this protocol every day in my office, I am excited that Ms. Bracco was brave enough to come out and say: You know, I wasn't feeling well, I was in a bad place, and I needed to do something about it and did! Not only did she do something about it, but she was so thrilled by the results, she wanted to share the news with the world. She has made a bold and innovative statement by doing this. *To the Fullest* has changed her life, has changed the lives of my patients, and will definitely change yours as well. Give it the best chance you can. Follow the program as if your life depends on it, because, frankly, it does.

FRED PESCATORE, MD,
AUTHOR OF THE BESTSELLER *THE HAMPTONS DIET*

A Work in Progress

Fifty . . . the F-word. That's how I saw it 10 years ago. My weight had been creeping up, and I had lost my sparkle. My energy and self-confidence were taking a dive. Everything was creaking. When I realized what was gradually happening to me, I made up my mind to transform myself. I wasn't ready to give up and free-fall into old age. It was time to put on the brakes and turn things around. I was ready to take charge of my life, to make the right choices so that I could be the best I could be every day. I'm a work in progress, and I'm not even close to being finished.

Too often we women are at the bottom of the list. Everyone else comes first. We are so busy looking after others—partners, husbands, boyfriends, children, aging parents, friends, colleagues, employees, and don't forget the pets—that we forget about what we need. We do everything for them and neglect ourselves. I had to focus more on myself if I wanted to stay healthy, lose weight, boost my energy, and feel terrific. I resolved to do everything I could to clean up my act.

My rejuvenation program began with making a commitment to take care of myself. **I realized that my body, mind, and spirit are the only things I really own. It was my responsibility to take care of what was mine. Since all three are adaptable, I had the power and the choice to change for the better. If I** wanted to stay vibrant and dynamic, I had to replace attitudes and habits that were depleting me with positive actions for change. *To the Fullest* is the story of what I did to come into my own and is a blueprint for rejuvenation. It would take a multifaceted program to achieve what I wanted.

I turned to three of my dear friends, Lisa Davis, Barbara King, and Monica Castellanos, for support. Lisa, an integrative health consultant, suggested that I try a liver cleanse. My response was, "Sure, why not?" Then she asked me, "Do you want to do a 'real' one or a 'cleanse lite'?"

I didn't hesitate to answer, "A real one!" Little did I know what I was getting myself into! I had never done any kind of cleanse before. I promised myself to do what I had to do to get back into shape. The cleanse was the perfect launch for my new, healthy approach to food and other life choices.

Following what I now call my Clean Up Your Act Plan, I set out to get rid of toxic buildup in my body that was affecting my health and making me sluggish, to break bad habits like my addiction to sugar, to eat well, and to move more. After consulting with my doctor, I cleaned my body from the inside out with an intensive liver cleanse. The 14-day cleanse I did is the core of *To the Fullest*.

Getting rid of toxins that had accumulated over the years was a solid start. Not only did I feel lighter and stronger after the cleanse, but I felt so good that changing the way I eat permanently was easy. It took me a year to lose the 35 pounds I had put on a little at a time and have kept that weight off for 4 years. I avoid processed food and almost anything in a package. I have become careful about the right way to eat. I haven't eaten gluten, sugar, or dairy since I began to jump-start change in my life. What may surprise you is that I never feel deprived.

Once I started to get myself back into shape, my spirits soared, my energy skyrocketed, and my confidence returned. I had it under control—it didn't have me! I can tell you that when you are feeling strong and healthy, you shine. I got my mojo back. Exercise became a pleasure, rather than a torment. Well, sometimes. I do know that exercise is another way to lift my spirits and make me glow. I feel the way I did decades ago, except I now have a greater understanding of what fulfills me. I'm happy in a way I've never been before. Okay, let's not get carried away—let's say that I'm comfortable in my own skin.

Friends, family, and fans on the street notice the change in me. They all do a double take when they see me and ask what I've done to myself. Everyone wants to know how I managed to come alive again. I've explained the steps I took to renew myself so often that I decided to write *To the Fullest* and get the word out.

I want more people—especially women—to benefit from what I have learned.

I would be less than honest if I neglected to say that Jimmy Gandolfini's shocking death contributed to my decision to motivate others to take care of themselves. I used to tease Jimmy about his expanding belly. He would pat it, smile, and say, "It's all muscle." The terrible, premature loss of a good friend and a talent, who was just coming into his own, was a jolting reminder of how vulnerable we are—here today and gone tomorrow. What a loss. You just can't take your health for granted.

I want to try to give you tools to slow down the aging process and prevent your body from breaking down and falling apart. **My goal is to inspire you to protect and restore your vitality, to be the best you can be at any age.** I especially want to help you live your life to the fullest from midlife and beyond. I want to share the program for change that worked for me and encourage you to break the bad habits that are undermining your health and the quality of your life.

You don't have to take just my word for it. As you read in Dr. Fred's foreword, volunteers completed the 2-week cleanse you will find in these pages and transitioned to the Clean Up Your Act Diet. The trial was a month for Dr. Pescatore's group and 6 weeks for the test group organized by Rodale, my publisher. The results for the Rodale group were phenomenal. Take a look at these numbers:

RESULTS AFTER 6 WEEKS ON THE PROGRAM

Most weight lost	16.8 pounds
Average weight lost	10.5 pounds
Most total inches lost	12 inches
Average total inches lost	8.4 inches
Most inches off arms	2 inches
Average inches off arms	1 inch
Most inches off chest	3 inches
Average inches off chest	1.4 inches
Most inches off waist	3.5 inches
Average inches off waist	2 inches
Most inches off hips	4.25 inches
Average inches off hips	1.7 inches
Most inches off thighs	3.75 inches
Average inches off thighs	2.2 inches

The weight and inches lost are only the outward signs of the benefits of the Clean Up Your Act Plan. I consider the weight loss a side effect. A lot more was going on inside the volunteers' bodies to improve their health. Lisa Davis, my BFF, has blood tests run before and after her clients do the cleanse. The tests have routinely shown a dramatic positive change in cholesterol and triglyceride levels.

The 14 wonderful women and one man who tried the cleanse that Rodale organized monitored their physical changes and recorded their reactions. At the start, they weren't feeling good and knew they needed to change. They were honest about what they found challenging in the program. I was moved by their enthusiasm and pride at what they had accomplished after 6 weeks on the plan. Their comments brought tears to my eyes. Their insights captured what happened to me as I took control of my life. Their words were so spot-on that I decided to include many of their comments throughout the book. Their experiences appear in Real Time Change sidebars. Their voices are as much a part of the book as mine. We are all in this together, after all.

If you only read the quotes from these women, you will see how powerful, focused, dedicated, and aware of themselves they were as they took back their lives. I've come to think of them as warriors for another life. Consider these Clean Up Your Act graduates a cheerleading squad. Their candid remarks will give you a realistic idea of what to expect, and their reports on how they changed will motivate you to stay with the program. Cleaning up our acts did wonders for all of us, and it will do the same for you.

Every day, you are exposed to poisonous chemicals in the air you breathe, the water you drink, the food you eat—processed food contaminated by countless chemical additives and conventionally raised produce, meat, and poultry full of hormones, antibiotics, genetically modified substances, pesticides, who knew?— the toxic household cleaning and personal grooming products you use, and from an endless array of damaging substances. Since I committed myself to living in a healthy way, I have made a study of how toxins affect us. I've read books, scholarly articles, the newsletters of environmental organizations, newspaper and magazine coverage, blogs. I've watched documentaries and lectures and talked to many experts to inform myself. I've immersed myself in learning about what in our environment has the potential to hurt us, the science behind the process of detoxification, and what we can do to reduce our toxic load. It's been quite an education! I've provided a list of selected sources in the back of the book, but they are just the tip of the iceberg. Between Lisa and me, we've got it covered. Trust me—the science in this book is backed by solid research. If you are interested in going deeper, look up anything you are curious about online. You'll find a wealth of information at your fingertips.

The program consists of a 14-Day Liver Cleanse that will begin to rid your body of the toxic load that has been building up over your lifetime. During the cleanse, you will have two protein shakes a day and take multivitamin/mineral and phytonutrient capsules to stimulate liver detoxification. We provide you with a list of the most effective supplements for your cleanse so you don't have to wander around the vitamin store to find effective products. There are so many choices it's confusing. You will eat a restricted diet during this time. The 2 weeks of meal plans and snacks I include will support your cleanse and make it deeper. These snacks and meals will prove to you that **hunger is not part of the program and eating clean has endless flavorful options.**

When you complete the cleanse, the Clean Up Your Act Diet prescribes a way to eat for the rest of your life. Your goal is to eat food that is close to the source. This is not one of those "magic bullet" deprivation diets on which you lose weight and soon gain it all back and more. I explain the benefits of eating gluten free, dairy free, and sugar free. Eating this way is not as challenging as you might think. First, you have to clean out that old junk in your kitchen cabinets. Get rid of it. Donate it to a charity that fights hunger or a senior center, or replace what you use gradually with healthy food. It's only taking up space and not doing you any good. I give you ideas for satisfying and delicious breakfasts, snacks, lunches, dinners, and desserts, along with shopping lists for the staples you will need for your new pantry—including delicious substitutes for the unhealthy, processed food you will no longer be tempted to eat. Since you are committing to a different way of eating, I've worked out 2 weeks of meal plans to help you get into it.

I love to cook, and that means whipping up a meal quickly. Who has time to prepare elaborate food these days? I may cook up a storm, but my style is no muss, no fuss. Since I vowed to clean up my act for good, I have changed the way I cook with health in mind. I will share some recipes that are as simple as they are tasty. With this healthy approach to eating every day, the pounds will steadily melt away and your energy will go through the roof. Good food changes everything. You will be rejuvenated on every level: Your skin will be radiant, those aches and pains will vanish, and your zest for life will be restored.

Moving is essential if you want to stay healthy. Not much will age you as quickly as being sedentary. I am not talking about working out so hard it hurts to walk the next day. I will show you how to make moderate exercise an enjoyable part of your life. Matt Natale, an integrative fitness and nutrition practitioner who has appeared on *The Biggest Loser,* has created three simple workouts for varying levels of fitness that you can do anywhere. Don't worry—I wouldn't let him work you to death. Whether you are a couch potato or a gym regular, one of these workouts is for you. As you get stronger, you can challenge yourself with a more demanding routine. **My goal is to win you over to the exercise habit, so that you will look forward to getting into your workout clothes.**

Finally, it is time for an attitude adjustment. **I want you to look at the rest of your life as a gift, not the beginning of the end. A lot can happen during your third act. You can reinvent your life if you want to.** Now you know what really matters to you. There is a freedom that comes with that knowledge. You can cut through the time-wasters and all the things that bring you down, make you angry, and stress you out, and go for what makes you happy. You will rise to life's challenges instead of throwing in the towel, because you're never too old to change.

To the Fullest will show you how to make healthy choices one step at a time. From diet to exercise, from self-acceptance to finding new passions, from keeping a sense of humor to doing the best you can each day, you will find all you need to start fresh in these pages. It is not too late to get back on track. You can reboot your body and set out on the path to vibrant health. **Just remember: The ability to live life to the fullest is ageless.**

To keep your motivation high and your commitment fresh, check out tothefullestbook.com, my interactive Web site. There you will find a support system that offers short videos on health, wellness, and inspiration, including diet, exercise, and topics ranging from meditation to growing a small organic garden. We'll answer your questions personally, give you seasonal recipes and meal plans so that you can enjoy the findings at your local farmers' market, and review and recommend healthy substitutes for processed food. Finding the most delicious treats I can eat is a never-ending quest for me! Believe me, I know the best gluten-free crackers and cookies on the market—I've tried them all. I got tired of bringing home bags of products that filled the bill nutritionally but tasted like cardboard. I started to sample the products right at the market. I'd stand in the aisle with my cart, tear open a box of cookies, and taste one. If I didn't like it, I threw the open package into my cart and paid for it with the rest of my groceries, but I didn't bother to take it home. I threw the product out at the cash register.

Recently, Lisa, Monica, and I went to a huge food expo at the convention center in Anaheim, California, and we must have had hundreds of samples during the weekend. The good news is that food manufacturers are making better and better prepared foods as we demand healthy choices. I've learned to read the nutrition labels on food and to study the ingredients and will tell you what to look for.

Through the Web site tothefullestbook.com, you will be in touch with a community of women who are making the same effort you are. You can turn to them for advice and moral support during the cleanse and for the broader issues that come with trying to age gracefully. I'm sure you will want to share your experiences and insights about sailing over the bumps in the road and to shine a light on the good things that lie ahead.

We are all in this together. **Remember: The only way to avoid aging is to die young.** It's time to enjoy the struggle. That's what living life to the fullest is all about.

LORRAINE BRACCO
JULY 2014

Above all, be the heroine of your life, not the victim.
—NORA EPHRON

CHAPTER

1

Wake-Up Call

Being part of *The Sopranos* was exhilarating. I was on top of the world. Depression, money problems, a brutal breakup and custody battle, and a failed business venture had brought me down, but all that was behind me. I had come out of a dark place and was stronger for it. I believed I had some good times ahead. My father kept my feet on the ground by reminding me that when Clark Gable—the King, the biggest star in the world—left the MGM lot for the last time, he walked through that gate alone and uncelebrated. It was my father's way of cautioning me that my success playing Dr. Melfi was transient. I'd been around long enough to know that, but working on the show did solve some pressing problems and freed me for some much-needed self-reflection. I was light-headed with relief!

I had raised my two daughters, Margaux and Stella, and worked hard to support them. By the time I turned 25, I had been a mother for a year. I had a little baby with a French father who was in love with someone else. I was so focused on getting by day-to-day that I never had a strategy for myself. I felt as

1

if I had been floundering from one thing to another my whole adult life. With the astronomical success of *The Sopranos,* I felt validated for the first time.

I finally could take a hard look and figure out what I had to do to get the most out of life rather than just struggling to survive. I did learn a lot along the way. I knew that life is never smooth sailing for long, but I believed in my heart of hearts I had lived through the worst. Nothing in my experience prepared me for the physical, emotional, and spiritual challenges in store for me.

The phrase "change of life" began to take on new meaning in my early fifties. I never believed hitting a certain age would make that much of a difference. I was who I was, and a dramatic shift wasn't going to happen to me. But it did. I had always been an eater, hungry all the time. I never stopped eating. Even so, weight hadn't been an issue. I was blessed with a hot and fast metabolism. When I hit 50, the metabolism I took for granted changed and the needle on the scale gradually started to move up. Getting dressed one morning, I stood there tugging on the zipper of my pants. I couldn't pull it up, no matter how much I sucked in my stomach. In denial, I raged through clenched teeth that the dry cleaner had shrunk the pants of my favorite suit. My answer to my increasingly tighter clothes was to tear out my hair.

REAL TIME CHANGE

Being a lifelong active, healthy woman, and someone who has always strived to lead a healthy lifestyle, I have noticed with the onset of menopause in the past 18 months, it has become more of a challenge to maintain as well as lose weight.

MARY LAMPE SUDDELL
NORTHPORT, NEW YORK

ME: You can say that again! Join the crowd. Nothing had prepared me for how much my body changed. I tried everything. Hormone replacement therapy didn't work for me. Messing with my hormones was not the answer.

There were other changes. I was famous for my ability to sleep anywhere, anytime. I could conk out on a park bench with five thousand people doing the samba around me. Suddenly, I had sleep problems. Not only did I have trouble getting solid sleep, but I was waking up with aches and pains. I got out of bed in stages. Sitting on the edge of the bed, I had to muster the energy to haul myself up to start the day, and I hadn't been partying the night before.

I have always loved wearing heels—the higher the better. I could never understand why women wore awful shoes as they got older, choosing comfort over style. But there I was, barely able to walk in my sexy shoes. The heavier I got, the harder it was. You have to be strong to wear high heels! Even though the pain was excruciating, I could not give them up—at least not for public appearances. Sensible shoes were not in the picture. I could manage to get from the car to my seat, where I would kick the shoes off with a sigh of relief and rest my tortured feet.

I was working to launch my wine company, Bracco Wines, and traveled all over the country wining and dining buyers. My weight continued to creep up. I was so busy I ignored what was happening to my body. It was easy to shrug off the changes. I would have time to deal with my weight, sleep deprivation, creaky body, and aching feet when things settled down. **One thing I have finally learned is that if you wait for things to calm down, you are talking about a long postponement, because it never happens. Life is not like that.** It's so easy to put off making a commitment to change. How many times have you said to yourself "next week" or "next month"? There are so many excuses for procrastinating—a New Year's resolution to start right after the holidays or when the kids go back to school

REAL TIME CHANGE

I teach full time, run three teenage boys around to their activities all evening, travel with my son's hockey team most weekends, and no longer take care of myself. I have gained 30 pounds in the past few years and feel completely out of shape and exhausted all the time. I need to put some focus back on me. This past year, I no longer feel healthy. I feel like I have aged tremendously. This year has been a big turning point in my health, and I can't get away with my current lifestyle.

STEPHANIE AUGELLO
BETHLEHEM, PENNSYLVANIA

ME: I'm so glad you had your hallelujah moment. If you don't take care of yourself, no one else will.

or when you finish that project at work. All I can say is that there's no time like right now.

The last episode of *The Sopranos* aired in June 2007. HBO served my wines at the finale party. Things were good for me. I was ready for an easy time with few worries. My two beautiful, intelligent daughters were out of the house and making their own way in the world. I am so proud of them. Margaux and Stella inspired me. They always make me want to be better. They were quick to comment on how I looked, critiquing my makeup and the clothes I wore.

At one point, they demanded I get out of the baggy sweats I lived in. They took me to a trendy store that sold a cute, young version of my wardrobe staple, made me buy some, and threw out the gross stuff I had been hanging out in. They nagged me about working out more. They didn't hold back. The tables had turned. My daughters were taking care of me. Watching them reminded me of how I used to be. I wanted to get some of that back.

Just as I was feeling liberated and open for anything, I was thrown into crisis mode. Early in 2008, both my parents became really sick, and the bottom dropped out of my world. My father, Sal, who had worked his whole life at the Fulton Fish Market, developed congestive heart failure. My mother, Sheila, a smoker, suffered a mild heart attack and battled emphysema. As my father said, their lives were about "pills and bills." Watching my parents' bodies fail them over a period of 3 to 4 years made it clear to me that aging is not for sissies. Seeing them suffer overwhelmed me. I was not ready for their decline.

And then there were the logistics of taking care of them. They were getting treatment at different hospitals. My brother, my sister, and I were running ourselves ragged racing from one appointment to another. I realize now that we have become a nation of caretakers. Not only do our adult children stay around longer, it took three of us to take care of our parents in their final years. Being their advocate and watching over them was a huge roller coaster ride. We were responsible for putting out fire after fire. It was very stressful, but I felt lucky I was able to be there for them. My parents had put up with so much from me as I grew up. They had been very open parents, and I loved them very much. Keeping them comfortable took precedence over everything else at the time. It was my turn to give to them.

Getting my father to be compliant was next to impossible. He never took his medication. I would organize what seemed like hundreds of colorful pills into his weekly pill sorter. He left the plastic organizer on the kitchen counter and completely ignored the schedule. He was so stubborn that I had Tony Sirico, the actor who played Paulie "Walnuts," give him a call. "Sal," he growled, "take your f***ing medicine!" My father was astonished but not threatened enough to gulp down all those pills. We did have some good laughs during their illnesses. The questionnaires we had to fill out at every new doctor's office became a running joke.

ME: Do you have a productive cough?

MOM (as she hacks up a lung): Absolutely not.

We tried our best to make their lives as normal as possible.

My parents died within 9 days of each other. Both were 84. They had been married for 64 years. I'm convinced that they chose to go out together. During their last few years, I was so focused on them that I never considered myself. I flew back and forth from Los Angeles to be with them in New Jersey. All I did was work, take care of them, and eat. I ignored my changing metabolism and didn't adjust my eating habits. I binged on old movies and two-pound bags of Twizzlers whenever I had time to collapse. For the first time in my life, I "needed" a drink at the end of the day. A little at a time, almost imperceptibly, my weight went up. **I gained more than 30 pounds in the time leading up to my parents' final illnesses. Their deaths were my wake-up call. It took losing my parents to make me realize I had to change my life to live it. What was I doing to myself?**

I wanted to be healthy. I did not want to be hooked up to oxygen like my mother. I did not want to take mountains of pills every day and live with the side effects. Crazy as it may seem, especially since my parents were so well taken care of, I became terrified of ending up helpless in a full-time care facility. **I could no longer afford to put off taking care of myself until it was too late. I needed a prevention and repair plan. If I did not commit to making changes in the way I lived, I could only go downhill.** I decided to do whatever it would take to stay healthy so that I could enjoy my two daughters and future grandchildren as long as I could. I was determined to stick around. I was not going to cave without a fight.

REAL TIME CHANGE

Trying the cleanse was a great opportunity at a time when I was just desperate to make life changes. I felt horrible. I ached all over. I had a full examination by my general practitioner, and he found nothing wrong. I just did not feel good. All of my joints ached. I was always tired and exhausted. I needed to fix myself but did not know how, and frankly, my doctor was no help at all.

I was in such a bad place—I was thinking, *God, send me a sign*, and he sent me Lorraine Bracco! God works in mysterious ways . . . and I am happier, healthier than I have been in forever. It is one of the best things I have ever done for myself. I am in full control of myself and in full control of my life. Who would have believed in 6 weeks I could totally transform myself? I really have!

LUCILLE IRCHA
NEW YORK, NEW YORK

ME: When a health care provider says, "Well, you're getting older—accept it," don't buy into it. It's so wrong. You don't have to accept feeling bad. You can always improve!

I cannot tell you how moved I was when I read this comment. The cleanse did the same for me. That's why I want to pass on what I've learned to other women who need to reboot their lives.

My hallelujah moment came when I watched my parents' health fail. So, I made a huge commitment to myself to take preventive action. I never had a problem with working hard. Now it was time to use that drive and energy on myself. I knew how easy it would be to lose my radiance and health in the years to come, to slip into dullness in body, mind, and spirit. I was ready to clean up my act and reclaim my life on my terms. I had to start with healing my body, which would have a ripple effect on my mental, emotional, and spiritual health. I had to make big changes in the way I lived.

Fortunately, my friend Lisa, who has spent her life as an integrative health consultant, had the answers. She encouraged me to jump-start change in my life by doing an intensive liver cleanse. She flew out to Los Angeles to do the cleanse

REAL TIME CHANGE

I was in a real slump in terms of identity. I like my job and am good at it. I love my family, and I think I give them my all and take good care of them. Still, there wasn't space for me in any of that, or rather, I'd not made space for me. I did not make time for myself, a crime I believe many mothers who work both inside and outside of the home commit. When I think of doing something for myself, I always think about learning a new skill or taking a class. Right before I signed on for the cleanse, though, I realized that work on me needed to start with me. I was ready to commit to myself, my well-being, and in turn, the well-being of my family. I needed to be the project.

MICHELE BLOOM
SOUTH ORANGE, NEW JERSEY

ME: You and the 14 others who did the cleanse for the Rodale trial had the same realization. I know how easy it is to lose yourself. We think of ourselves last. Focusing on yourself and making your health a priority is the first step to being the best you can be.

with me. It probably couldn't have been a worse time, because I was starting the second season of *Rizzoli & Isles* and had just rented an empty house that I had to move into, set up, and furnish. But it was also the perfect time, because I was completely committed to doing the cleanse, so what better way to start than with an empty fridge and pantry—no temptations to toss out, just a clean slate. And so began my new journey.

As someone who never had to think too much about what I ate, I expected to suffer following a diet that seemed very restrictive to me. I can honestly say that after the 2-day fast that kicks off the program, it was a breeze. I felt and saw the results of this new way of eating so quickly that I wasn't even tempted to revert to my old ways. I'm not saying that I lost a pound a day. My weight loss was slow and steady. Sure, I hit plateaus, but I toughed it out and continued to lose.

Eating clean has become a way of life for me. Once I figured out what my foods could or should be, I never turned back. I knew this is what I had to do, what I wanted to do. As I said earlier, I love to eat. In fact, I turn ferocious when

I'm hungry. "Did we feed the beast?" is often asked when I arrive on set. I am happy to report that I don't have to go hungry to eat well on the Clean Up Your Act Diet. **When I am tempted to eat candy or a piece of bread, I look at the temptation in front of me and ask, "What are you going to do for me?" I already know the answer: "Nothing good." Stopping to remind myself of that helps to build my resistance to the empty, dead foods I thought I couldn't live without. Now I want to eat food that gives to me rather than takes away.** I make conscious choices about what I put in my mouth. "Comfort food" has become food that really nourishes me, giving me sustained energy and dense nutrition.

That is not to say I'm always perfect. When I do break the rules, I choose to do so. Every Saturday night in Los Angeles, I have two lychee martinis at one of my favorite restaurants and enjoy every sip. I look forward to it all week! Whenever I return to New York from Los Angeles, I have to have a slice of pizza. I'm not a fanatic at holidays. I'm not going to skip my mother's ricotta balls, which she learned to make from my grandmother and which I in turn make every Christmas for my children. But Thanksgiving or Christmas dinner is just one meal on one day, not a season of overeating all the wrong food. I do make a conscious choice to stray from eating clean now and then, but I enjoy indulging in overly sweet, starchy food less and less. It just doesn't feel good to eat that way anymore.

Along the path of rejuvenation, I started looking at myself and the world differently. Negative thinking was out. Right before David Chase approached me about joining the cast of *The Sopranos*, I was emotionally and financially bankrupt. A vicious, 10-year custody battle had left me clinically depressed. I was lost for a year before I did anything to pull out of it. During that dark time, I read a lot and gained an understanding of a deeper side of life. As bleak as depression was, I grew so much from going through it. This time of reflection gave me a fuller sense of who I was and what mattered to me. Glamour, success, celebrity are all great, but what has lasting value and matters most to me is far more simple and lasting—family, health, and a good laugh.

After I got medical help, the dark cloud lifted, and I was able to see that the window had always been open. I flew out of that prison. Nothing could make me go back. What was splendid in the world around me became a constant source of joy. I had a new appreciation of how rich downtime could be.

So that's the story of my transformation. I am about to turn 60 as I write this book. I now have a breathtaking granddaughter named Vivienne. I can't get enough of her. I am at the top of my game. And I can wear stilettos again without hobbling in pain! As my birthday approaches, I keep saying to myself, "Hello 60!" I plan to have the best decade yet. I'm 60, and I can still turn a head! I want you to know that it's not too late. Change is within your reach. It's easier than you think. Just read on.

We are taught you must blame your father, your sisters, your brothers, the school, the teachers—but never blame yourself. It's never your fault. But it's always your fault, because if you wanted to change, you're the one who has got to change.

—KATHARINE HEPBURN

CHAPTER

2

Love the Struggle

From the time I was 17 to when I turned 27, I lived in Paris where I worked as a model. Wilhelmina Models agency had sent me for a monthlong assignment. After a café au lait and a croissant on my first morning, I fell in love with the city and stayed for 10 years. I modeled, worked as a producer in French TV, acted in several European films, and hosted a radio talk show for Radio Luxembourg during that time. You have to understand that I was voted the ugliest girl on the bus in sixth grade—a title I've never really gotten over. Modeling in Paris and acting in foreign movies were far from what I ever expected to do. A high school teacher had seen something in me and helped me break into modeling. I couldn't believe my luck! I never thought I deserved it, but I dove right in and ran with it. And I never looked back.

I learned so much about style and attitude by observing French women in my formative years. French women understand what happens to them at 35, 45,

55. They are not done in by aging. They accept themselves and highlight their best qualities. They value the wisdom and savvy they have accumulated. **French women know that confidence and passion for living makes a woman—or anyone for that matter—appealing at any age.** I'm not saying that they sit back and let time take its toll. They are minutely self-aware. They have mastered maintenance and are always considering ways to improve their appearance. From shop girls to women of a certain age, they have a unique elegance and know how to put themselves together to be chic and striking. They do not believe their appeal fades as they age. They never stop trying to be alluring. They are sexy until they die.

They do stay thin and wear their clothing well. As I observed them in cafes, restaurants, at parties, and in their homes, they didn't seem to deprive themselves of fine food and all that butter, cream, and cheese. **French women are brilliant at portion control. They know when to put their forks down. They use a system of checks and balances and rarely overindulge.** If they eat cheese, bread, and wine at a meal, they skip the pastries for dessert and have fruit with a cup of espresso. It's all about balance and control. I couldn't have had better role models.

Eating processed food was not an option for them. The French eat close to the source. Since France is a small country, shipping food from where it is raised or caught to anywhere in the country doesn't take very long. Everything they eat is fairly fresh. There are open markets around every corner. You don't have to go far to find clean food to eat. The same was true of most of Europe. I spent some time in a little town in Tuscany a few years ago. Fish or seafood was not on the menu of a single restaurant in town. I asked one owner why that was. With a shrug of his shoulders, he answered, "The sea is 3 hours away." The people of the village were still eating what was produced locally as their ancestors did centuries ago. Their cuisine was built around what was found in the region. Fortunately, truffles were one of the local "crops."

Only until very recently, processed food was just not available in France. I am sorry to say that there is now a McDonald's in the Louvre. I've read that hamburgers have become the current food fad in France. Globalization seems to be changing the way Europeans eat, not for the good. But I bet when a chic French woman eats a hamburger and fries, she skips the bun, only picks at the fries, and makes sure she has a salad or fruit!

It's interesting that the "locavore" and farm-to-table movements in the United States are on an upswing as the rest of the world adopts our less-than-healthy eating habits. We know the effect that fast food and highly processed food has had on us—two out of three people in this country are overweight. Since the 1950s, we have been gorging ourselves on processed food with little nutritional value, and we are exporting obesity to the rest of the world. I'm excited by the movement here to get back to eating clean, fresh food. It's definitely a giant step in the right direction.

There's nothing I love more than wandering through the farmers' markets in Los Angeles and New York. Taking in all the colors and smells makes me happy. Preparing and eating the delicious ingredients I find is even better. The reason I digress is that a diet of fresh food keeps you healthier longer, which certainly contributes positively to your appearance and state of mind.

The European attitude about aging recognizes the value of mellowing with the passage of time. Beauty is not judged just by an unlined face and a perfect body. Inner qualities of assurance, sophistication, grace, and charm count for a lot. **Recognizing the changes in their bodies, French women make the effort to look as good as they can and to have style whatever their age. They never give up trying to be attractive. They still feel desirable, because European culture does not dismiss women once they hit their forties.**

Youth is everything here in the United States. It's easy to think that you're over the hill, that you've reached your expiration date, when the standard of beauty is based on being young. You're considered seriously over the hill once you approach 50. In Los Angeles, the cut-off date begins at 35. I see so many people, especially in my line of work, who are cosmetic surgery addicts, trying to stop or turn back the clock. The pressure is so intense that men and women are starting earlier and earlier to revise their faces and bodies. They strive to achieve a vision of perfection, and many lose a sense of where they started. I don't know what they see when they look in the mirror. Aside from a frightening addiction to cosmetic surgery, they smoke to keep their weight down and starve themselves all day only to binge on a bag of chips or cookies for dinner. Have you ever noticed that people eat too little or too much? Rarely does anyone hit the right balance. The choices the young people are making will catch up with them and ruin the looks they are trying so hard to preserve. More importantly, they are putting their health in jeopardy.

Personally, I would never go for such a dramatic change in my appearance. To paraphrase Coco Chanel, I've earned the face I have! I do take very good care of my skin and try the latest treatments to keep it looking fresh and tight, but I'm not interested in major alterations. **In the end, I want to *feel* like I'm 25, not look that age.**

YOU DON'T HAVE TO BECOME INVISIBLE

In our society, women become invisible when they hit middle age. Everyone suddenly calls you "ma'am." The waiter stops flirting with you. Sales clerks just look past you as if you don't exist. The cashier at the movie theater asks if you want senior tickets years before you qualify. People start to offer you a seat on the subway without making eye contact. Cab drivers no longer help you with packages, and attendants don't show you the way to your seat at a ball game. These small slights and so many like them make you cringe inside. You might pass a mirror or see your reflection in a store window and not recognize yourself, thinking, "Who's that old woman?" You begin to feel as if you are vanishing.

If you're crying just about now, get a grip, sister. We've all been there. When the world responds to you with disinterest, the message is that you are no longer vital, important, or remarkable.

The feeling that you are not worth noticing doesn't do a lot for your self-esteem. It's no surprise that so many women just give up. Why bother to take good care of yourself when you are resigned to a life sentence of invisibility? You can begin to believe that you don't deserve the best. Giving up, you pile on the pounds, stop exercising, delay getting your roots done, pull your hair back with a scrunchie or cut it all off, and resort to loose clothes and gym shoes. The message that you are sending is that you do not value yourself enough to make the most of who you are. Nothing will make you disappear from view faster.

Stop fading away. You can choose not to go along with being pushed into the background. You can reclaim your body and your mind and become visible again. Being down on yourself doesn't help you to change. You have to accept yourself and take responsibility for who you are. If you look in the mirror and sigh, thinking, "I'm overweight, old, and boring. Aging is the worst," that is who you are. If you think, "I used to have a tiny waist. Now look at me, I'm hopeless," living in the past is not doing you any good. You have to live in the moment and not measure yourself against an image of yourself that is decades old. And while you're at it, don't take yourself so seriously. Being able to laugh at and even appreciate your supposed "flaws" will make them easier to live with. I don't love my stretch marks and the little stomach pooch that won't go away whatever I do, but I view them as well-earned achievement badges from my pregnancies. They are a small price to pay for having brought the daughters I adore into the world.

Being truthful to yourself is not always easy, especially after years of avoidance. It's time to take a close look at yourself and commit to changing what you do not like. It's all about the choices you make. You will either reap the benefits or suffer the consequences. By the way, there's nothing uglier than bitterness. You have the power to make choices that will enhance your feelings of self-worth. Make a commitment to treat yourself with the respect and love you show others. As you evaluate yourself right now, you can say, "I'm not so bad, but we can all be better. I can be more than what I am today." You do not have to stagnate. **There is no reason to stop trying. You deserve to be a priority.**

EMBRACE CHANGE

Nothing stays the same in life—both the good and the bad. You have to embrace change; otherwise you will be stuck in a time warp. Thinking of all that is new in the world in my lifetime fills me with awe. It's hard to imagine life without cell phones, texting, e-mail, the Internet, or Netflix. It takes energy to keep up, but why be left behind when so much is happening?

Yes, you are different from how you were in your twenties, and you will continue to change. **Inside of you is a blueprint of the best you can be at any given age, a template of what is perfect for you.** You can work to improve what you don't like about yourself. There is so much you can do to put on the brakes to slow the pace of aging. This is your chance to begin a new life. Set some realistic goals and go for it. No one else will do it for you. Accept that it will take time and effort to reach those goals. The Clean Up Your Act Plan will help you to kick-start positive change. **The truth is that you have to learn to love the struggle—that's what life is all about. Nothing comes easy, but it's so rewarding to succeed.** There is nothing holding you back but yourself. You have one life. Why not make the most of it?

People in their twenties and thirties are all beautiful to me now. Their looks do all the talking. The atmosphere around them is intense, flirtatious, and competitive. Once you approach 50, you are no longer considered in the game, which is one of the reasons you may feel as if you have disappeared. If you look at the situation from a different angle, not being a player can be very liberating. Since you have nothing to lose, you can say whatever you want to whomever you want. You don't have to play by the rules. You can become an outrageous older woman, who does not hesitate to say what she thinks to anyone, delivered with a big smile, disarming wit, and charm. You will be surprised how easy it is to win people over if you are open, outgoing, and just a bit bigger than life. You will not stay disappeared for long.

A friend and I were enjoying lunch on the terrace of a restaurant overlooking the Pacific on a perfect, sunny day. I found my eye drawn to a table of women nearby. I couldn't tell how old they were or whether they were younger or older than I. As I've explained, guessing someone's age can be hard in Los Angeles these days. They were all attractive but dull—nothing was coming off them. There they were on a gorgeous day, drinking wine, and chatting, but they were not shining, brilliant, or exciting. It was as if the light had been turned off inside them. They had lost their edge, and I wondered what had happened. Where were they? And then I realized that had been me.

I wanted to go up to them and shake them alive. Being a vibrant, powerful presence was still within the reach of every one of those women. I could have been just like them if I hadn't taken a leap and decided not to give up on myself.

When I set to work on my self-renewal program, my daughter Margaux, who is wise beyond her years, gave me some good advice. "Every night when you go to bed," she said, "ask yourself if you did the best you could today." I still ask myself that question every night and will until my last. **Demanding the best from yourself in any circumstance is what loving the struggle is all about. You have it in you to shine and to rise above the forces of time that are constantly working to break you down. Enjoy the challenge!**

In the next chapter, I examine the hunger within each of us that is usually based on self-doubt or dissatisfaction. I want you to discover what moves your soul and what will expand your imagination about the possibilities in your life.

To laugh often and much; to win the respect of intelligent people and the affection of children; to earn the appreciation of honest critics and endure the betrayal of false friends; to appreciate beauty; to find the best in others; to leave the world a bit better, whether by a healthy child, a garden patch or a redeemed social condition; to know even one life has breathed easier because you have lived. This is to have succeeded.

—RALPH WALDO EMERSON

I'm selfish, impatient and a little insecure. I make mistakes. I am out of control and at times hard to handle. But if you can't handle me at my worst, then you sure as hell don't deserve me at my best.

—MARILYN MONROE

CHAPTER

3

The Hunger Within

Looking back, I realize that an emptiness inside drove me to find comfort in food during the stressful period leading to my parents' illnesses. My overeating coincided with a changing metabolism brought about by menopause—a formula for disaster! Food was one of my only pleasures. I can't tell you how much I looked forward to falling into bed to watch a movie and treat myself to tons of candy at the end of an exhausting day. Powerful emotions were triggering my eating. I wasn't even hungry. I was eating to blunt those feelings. Bingeing on

17

sweet, fatty foods distracted me from what was happening in my life. Comfort food only offered temporary relief from the demands of the moment. It became a self-defeating cycle: My emotions triggered me to overeat, then I felt miserable because I couldn't get into any of my clothes. When I was down on myself, I would reach for a bag of licorice to feel better. What a trap! I began to hate my body. That negativity did not inspire me to make long-lasting changes.

GETTING A HANDLE ON EMOTIONAL EATING

Each one of us has a hunger within that is usually based on self-doubt, self-loathing, or dissatisfaction. Some of us accumulate things to satisfy that hunger. When I started working on *Rizzoli & Isles*, I rented a beautiful house in Beverly Hills, which I filled up with so much stuff. It took me no time at all. Recently, I bought a gem of a house in the hills that has a beautiful view of the city. It's a little bit of magic. It felt great to get rid of everything I had managed to collect and to simplify the place where I live. All those things had nothing to do with my happiness. What mattered was the good times I had in the house, not the things I had acquired. I feel so much lighter without all of it!

Sometimes we attempt to fill the emptiness inside with food, which offers temporary satisfaction until the consequences come. You probably already know what unhealthy food you crave when you are stressed out, angry, fearful, sad, lonely, or bored. **Chronic stress physically triggers cravings for the terrible trio: salty, sweet, and fatty foods.** Whether ice cream, cookies, chips, or pizza, we use food in our culture to deal with our feelings. We see a visual of this behavior in every movie or TV show that features a depressed, disappointed, anxious, or lonely woman of any age. Eating can literally be a way of "stuffing down" uncomfortable emotions. **Numbing yourself with food enables you to avoid emotions you'd rather not feel**. When you feel unfulfilled, empty, and bored, food can be a way to fill you up and distract you from the dissatisfaction with your life. By the way, there is no difference between food, drugs, sex, booze, and shopping—all of these will numb you.

We use food as a reward. Think of the treats you received when you were a kid—an ice-cream cone after a school performance, a lollipop at the doctor's office, a home-baked cookie to cheer you up when you were sad or disappointed. You learned to push away feelings with a treat as a child, and if you are like me, you carried that way of coping into adulthood.

Emotions in Traditional Chinese Medicine

In traditional Chinese medicine, the seven basic emotions—anger, sadness, worry, pensiveness, fear, shock (fright), and joy—are associated with specific organs. Each organ has a corresponding emotion. An imbalance of a particular emotion over a period of time affects how the organ functions. It goes the other way, too. A diseased or imbalanced organ can produce symptoms of the emotion related to it. I find this system of mind-body connection fascinating. The system underscores the importance of learning to deal with your emotions if you want optimal health and well-being. Otherwise, suppressed emotions will play out in your body.

You should keep the intimate connection between your emotions and organs in mind when you examine the way you respond to the challenges in your life. What you are feeling has a direct effect on your health in this ancient Chinese system. One of the reasons I've included this information is that some of the symptoms you experience while your body is detoxifying could indicate where imbalances are located. Here is a breakdown:

Anger-Liver
Anger can take the form of resentment, bitterness, frustration, irritability, and explosiveness. Symptoms of liver imbalance include lumps in the breast, menstrual pain, headache, dizziness, tendonitis, dry, red eyes and other eye conditions.

Sadness-Lungs
Sadness includes grief and detachment. Imbalance in the lungs can produce fatigue, shallow breathing, sweating, a cough, frequent colds and flu, allergies, asthma, dry skin, depression, and crying.

Worry-Spleen
In our stressed-out society, worrying is common. When worry or anxiety depletes the energy of the spleen, digestive disturbances and chronic fatigue can develop. Symptoms of an imbalanced spleen include: loss of appetite, poor digestion, abdominal bloating, diarrhea, weak muscles, pale lips, excessive menstrual bleeding, and bruising.

Pensiveness-Spleen
Pensiveness is also identified as concentration, obsessing about a topic, thinking too much, or excessive mental and intellectual stimulation. An

(continued)

Emotions in Traditional Chinese Medicine—Continued

imbalance in the spleen causes worry, resulting in fatigue, lethargy, and inability to concentrate. Symptoms exhibited are poor appetite, bloating after eating, and paleness.

Fear-Kidneys

Other emotions considered to be aspects of fear are insecurity, isolation, aloofness, and weak willpower. A kidney imbalance can lead to frequent urination or incontinence, dry mouth, poor short-term memory, night sweats, low back pain, hearing loss, ringing in the ears, osteoporosis, premature gray hair, and hair loss.

Shock-Heart and Kidneys

Shock or fright is distinguished from fear by its sudden, unexpected nature. Fright primarily affects the heart in the initial stages, but if it persists it becomes fear and moves to the kidneys. The heart responds with palpitations, anxiety, and insomnia. The fight-or-flight reaction causes an excess of adrenaline to be produced from the adrenal gland that sits on the kidney. If the stress is chronic, the kidney is affected.

Joy-Heart

A disorder related to joy might be surprising. Don't we all want as much joy in our lives as possible? In Chinese traditional medicine, joy refers to states of agitation or overexcitement rather than deep contentment. Even good news can be stressful. If you are on overdrive and live a life of excess, you can develop heart imbalances with palpitations, anxiety, and insomnia.

Your emotions have a powerful effect on your body and health. When you tamp down those emotions by distracting yourself with food, you will throw your body off balance and eventually undermine your health.

We also celebrate by feasting. Think of all the blow-out events like weddings, birthdays, anniversaries, graduation parties, and holidays, when it's hard to refrain from eating too much of the wrong foods. Your social life probably revolves around eating specially prepared meals or at restaurants with family and friends. What you have to remember is that it's about the company, not the food. You can still celebrate and eat in a healthy way.

When you do the 14-Day Liver Cleanse and follow it up by making the healthy food choices of the Clean Up Your Act Diet, you will break your pattern of emotional eating, because what you can and cannot eat is very specific. You are in control. I can tell you it feels good. If you want to make the healthy changes in your diet permanent, you have to understand what is behind your cravings for junk food. If you don't look at why you overeat, swearing off the unhealthy food you crave will probably not last for long. If you have gone on a crash diet, lost weight, and gained it right back, you know what I'm talking about. Willpower alone won't do it. You have to deal with the psychological and spiritual dimension of the problem.

REAL TIME CHANGE

My biggest obstacle to making healthy changes: emotional eating. I eat to numb and distract.

DIANE ARPINO
RAMSEY, NEW JERSEY

ME: Eating can be a form of self-medicating, and numbing is a habit that easily can become an addiction. That's why dealing with your emotions head-on and learning what triggers your cravings is so important. Even though it's much harder to feel, I'd rather feel than be numb any day.

BREAKING UP WITH COMPULSIVE EATING

Identifying what triggers your emotional eating is the first step in breaking free from food cravings and compulsive eating. It helps to keep a Mood and Food journal to record when and where you had an urge to eat, what triggered the impulse, what you ate, and how you felt before and after. You should assess how hungry you were on a scale of 1 to 10. If your hunger was 6 or above, you probably were physically hungry; below 5 on the scale indicates you are driven to eat for reasons other than hunger. Separating hunger from just wanting to eat is an important distinction. Keeping this sort of record will make you aware of a pattern in your behavior that will help you to overcome mindless eating.

Emotional eating is automatic and unconscious. Rather than reaching for your fix, pause for a minute and think about why you want to eat. Waiting just a

REAL TIME CHANGE

I had to frost cupcakes for my daughter's birthday party at school, and I realized how thoughtlessly I eat broken pieces of cupcakes and how frequently I "check" the frosting. During the cleanse, I didn't crave anything but would have eaten whatever was put in front of me. I realize how much during the day I just eat because something is in front of me. Life Lesson 5.

MICHELE BLOOM
SOUTH ORANGE, NEW JESEY

ME: Being mindful about what you eat changes everything. Nothing goes in my mouth unless I make a conscious decision to have it. Taking control of my eating gave me such a sense of power, which carried over to every aspect of my life. I feel as if I own my actions, and it's great!

minute can give you the awareness to make a different food choice. While you are at it, take a moment to allow yourself to feel the emotion behind the craving. Accept what you are feeling without judgment. Experiencing the emotion will help you to understand your deepest fears, desires, and frustrations and point you toward what will make you happy. So what's wrong with a good cry or feeling sad or angry? These are healthy things. **Don't hold on to appropriate emotions. Facing your feelings will make them subside quickly. I don't know why we run away from our feelings. Emotions add great texture to life. Being open to your emotional responses will keep you connected moment by moment to the present. Being in the moment will enrich your life immeasurably.**

You might want to try a simple calming breath technique. Close your eyes. Inhale deeply and slowly to a count of 10, hold your breath for a moment, then exhale to a count of 10. Repeat this six times. Observe the thoughts as they surface in your mind and let them float by without responding or analyzing. In a little more than 2 minutes, you will find yourself calmer.

On a practical note, it takes effort to binge if you have to leave the house to buy what you crave. Clean out your cupboards and refrigerator and dump all the junk food that is not good for you. No hidden stashes of candy or chips allowed. You should always have healthy snacks on hand. Check out the list of my go-to treats on page 143.

FIND OTHER MOOD BOOSTERS

You have to find ways to give yourself a quick pick-me-up that don't have caffeine or calories. Feed your mind. I love to watch documentaries, because they shine a light on what is going on in the world. I can binge-watch five in a sitting! Read, listen to music, connect with nature. Doing any of these things will make you feel better than eating comfort food that isn't good for you. You can make a cup of tea. If you're depressed, call a cheerful friend or watch your favorite sitcom. Turn on music and dance when you're anxious. Exercise is a cure-all. Not only does moving burn up the excess energy produced by worry and fear, but it also creates energy when you are down. You have to expend energy to have energy. You can always take a soothing bath or read a magazine or book. Better yet, do them both at the same time. You can make your bath more luxurious by adding a few drops of an essential oil with healing properties.

Having alternatives to mindless bingeing that you can fall back on will help you overcome the impulse to pig out on junk food. Taking the time to relax can be a big help. So many of us feel there's something wrong with simply doing nothing. We work hard to achieve what we want and forget to treat ourselves to downtime for rest and relaxation. You need to de-stress regularly. Instead of reaching for a snack that fails to satisfy in the long run, it makes sense to do something that will lift your mood and make you feel good inside.

THE FOUR-BITE RULE

If you just can't resist the temptation of a sinful indulgence, limit what you eat to four bites. You don't have to eat the whole candy bar, bag of chips, or pint of ice cream. Moderation is the answer. I read somewhere that your memory of food is limited to the first four bites. A week later, you will remember those four bites of flourless chocolate cake as just as good an experience as downing the whole slice. **If you stop your indulgence after a few bites, you'll get the same short-lived pleasure at a lower cost.** I have some friends who always serve an amazing chocolate cake at their Fourth of July party. I don't even try to resist it—it's that delicious. I take a couple of bites and let them melt in my mouth. That's enough for me. It doesn't get better than those first few bites!

Essential Oils and the Emotions They Ease

I love soaking in a fragrant, steamy bath. Aside from being a sensual pleasure, natural essential oils have potent healing properties. Aromatherapy can be a big help when you are confronting difficult or painful emotions. Only a few drops are needed at a time. Their molecules are very small, so they can be easily absorbed by the skin to do their work. A small bottle can last a few years if you use the oil sparingly. Citrus oils lose their potency after 2 years, but most have a shelf life of 5 to 10 years.

TO EASE	TRY
Anger	Chamomile, jasmine, marjoram, rose, rosemary, ylang-ylang
Anxiety	Bergamot, chamomile, frankincense, geranium (for balance), lavender, orange, patchouli, rose (for confidence), sandalwood, sweet marjoram, vetiver (for grounding)
Disappointment	Bergamot, cypress, frankincense, jasmine, orange, rose
Fatigue(emotional and mental)	Basil, cardamom, cinnamon leaf or bark, clove bud, coriander, eucalyptus, ginger, grapefruit, jasmine, juniper, orange, peppermint, rosemary, thyme, vetiver, ylang-ylang
Fatigue (physical)	Basil, ginger, lemon, lavender, orange, peppermint, rosemary
Fear	Cedarwood, fennel, ginger, patchouli, sandalwood, thyme
Grief	Bergamot, chamomile, jasmine, marjoram, rose
Hysteria	Chamomile, lavender, orange, tea tree
Impatience	Chamomile, frankincense, lavender
Indecision	Basil, cypress, jasmine, patchouli, peppermint
Jealousy	Jasmine, rose
Loneliness	Benzoin, marjoram
Nervousness	Chamomile, coriander, frankincense, orange, vetiver
Panic	Chamomile, geranium, jasmine, juniper, lavender, ylang-ylang
Sadness	Jasmine, rose, rosewood

Shock	Lavender, rose, tea tree
Shyness	Black pepper, ginger, jasmine, patchouli, peppermint, rose, ylang-ylang
Stress	Bergamot, Atlas cedarwood, Roman chamomile, all citrus oils, sage, frankincense, geranium, lavender, sweet marjoram, patchouli, rose, rosemary, sandalwood, vetiver, and ylang-ylang
Suspicion	Jasmine, lavender
Tension	Chamomile, cypress, frankincense, geranium, jasmine, lavender, lemon, marjoram, orange, rose, rosewood, sandalwood, ylang-ylang

This chart has been adapted from "Oils That Can Ease Unpleasant Emotions: Emotional Effects of Aromatherapy" on naturesgift.com/emotbl.htm.

This list is limited to the most accessible oils. I have an oil for every mood and occasion, and I love to mix them. I confess that I don't like the scent of lavender, but I have included it because so many people find it soothing. We forget how powerfully scent shapes our moods. For me, there is nothing like the smell of clean laundry or, even better, my baby granddaughter.

DON'T WAIT TO BOTTOM OUT

I've noticed that hitting rock bottom, suffering a terrible loss, or any number of catastrophes is often what sparks a spiritual awakening. Feeling as if you have experienced the worst can free you and clarify your priorities. A crisis can give you the insight and drive to change, as it did for me. People wait until they are so sick that they are on their knees begging God to help them, promising "I won't smoke" or "I won't drink anymore."

I had an on-my-knees moment when Stella was 9. I was attending the Sundance Film Festival for *Basketball Diaries*, which starred Leonardo diCaprio before he made *Titanic*. That adorable young man chose me to play his mother. Doing the film was a great experience for me as an actor. I had only four lines, but we made it into something. This small role received fantastic reviews. I was thrilled to go to Sundance with a good film and was happy to take the 10-hour trip through Salt Lake City to Park City, Utah.

I was there maybe 10 minutes when I got a call from the woman who was taking care of the girls while I was away. She told me I needed to get home immediately—something was wrong with Stella. My mother got on the phone and explained that Stella was running an extremely high temperature and was terribly sick. The urgency I heard in their voices prompted me to turn around and get home as soon as I could.

Stella had seen her pediatrician by the time I arrived home, and he had begun running blood tests. I found her glassy-eyed and very lethargic with a fever of 104 to 105 degrees. She stayed home from school for 2 weeks, and the fevers kept on coming. After I gave her aspirin and her fever went down, she was so chilled that she would shake all over. I couldn't keep her warm. I'd cover her with a doubled-up silk blanket someone had given me as a gift and would use my body to try to warm her up. This went on for 2 weeks, until her pediatrician referred us to specialists.

I have nothing but praise for the doctors at Mount Sinai. They went through a process of elimination, first checking for cancers such as leukemia or lymphoma. I stayed at the hospital with her through all of this. They did so many tests—spinal taps, PET scans—it seemed so invasive. It was such a difficult time—I would go out in the hall and scream, "You have to find out what this is!" Waiting for the diagnosis was unendurable. I was losing my mind with worry.

One day, a nurse took the thermometer out of Stella's mouth, looked shocked,

REAL TIME CHANGE

I turned 55 this year and have not only struggled with my weight in recent years but felt my energy level had much to be desired. My children are now in their early twenties and "almost" out of the house. It's time for me to enter into a new phase of my life, and I wanted to be at my best as they also enter into adulthood.

LORETTA LANG STOKES
BEVERLY, MASSACHUSETTS

ME: Once the kids are gone, you don't want to be a sick old lady. This is your time to enjoy your life. You are free! Believe me, the new phase of your life can be the best ever. Cleaning up your act now will make all the difference. Be the best you can be!

shook the thermometer, looked again, and started to walk away. "It must be broken," she said.

I was frantic, "What did it say?"

"107 degrees—it's not possible. I'm going to get a thermometer that works."

"Don't even think of leaving her." I was in a panic. "Do something; do anything to bring her fever down." She knew I was serious. I was like a mother bear protecting her cub.

Until they learned what was wrong, I was terrified that I would lose her. I got down on my knees and prayed to God not to take my daughter, to take this illness away. I implored God to make me sick instead. I've had many drop-to-my-knees moments—to pay the mortgage, to get a part, to find someone to love me and not be alone—but on my knees for Stella was by far the hardest moment of my life. I felt completely alone.

After going through every test known to man, Stella was diagnosed with an autoimmune disease, juvenile rheumatoid arthritis. Knowing what was wrong was a relief—it could have been so much worse. Until the time she was 16 or 17, she had several bouts that began with a high fever and a strep infection. Her joints would get stiff and painful during a flare-up, but she grew out of it.

I will always remember praying desperately to God to save her. It was a turning point. I learned in a very visceral way that without your health you have nothing. That lesson made me aware of the importance of prevention.

The fact is, you can think about how you want to lead your life anytime. Why wait for disaster? **Don't wait until you have stage 4 cancer to be motivated to change. You can put your energy into prevention at any time.**

Though the ability to change is always with you, you can get caught up in the demands of your day-to-day life. That preoccupation can distance you from what would profoundly move your soul and enhance your feeling of well-being. The days fly by in a flash of work, chores, and countless things you have to do. You're always thinking about what's next on the list. If you don't carve out time for yourself to enrich your life or simply unwind, you will miss so much of what life has to offer.

LIGHTEN UP

You are taking an important step by clearing your body of toxins and nourishing it with wholesome, healing food. **When your body is well nourished and work-**

ing at its best, your mind and emotions are no longer dragged down. As you are cleansing your body, you have to detoxify your mind. Your thoughts and feelings are so powerful that negativity affects your entire body. Feelings of judgment, anger, and hate will take their toll on you. They eat you up inside and show externally on your face and body. You become what you are thinking. If you look in the mirror and think, "I am ugly, fat, and have done nothing with my life," that is exactly what you project. Energy follows thought. When you think, "I'm sick and tired. There's nothing left for me to live for," you will make that judgment right, even though you are wrong.

Good thoughts and an optimistic attitude will bring light into your life. Being generous in your actions and thoughts will open up the world to you. Just as you commit to cleaning up your act when it comes to diet, do the same with your state of mind. I think that I have the whole, wide world ahead. It's the last third of my life, and I intend to enjoy it. In fact, it's going to be the best time of my life.

The simple deep-breathing meditation I described on page 22 can make you aware of the emotional ruts in which your mind gets stuck. Watching what is going on in your head without judgment or trying to deal with it is a way to separate yourself from those intense feelings and to make room for your natural inner peace to surface. Sit in a comfortable chair in a quiet place without too many distractions. That means turn off the TV. I am so used to leaving the TV on as background noise. When I have to learn lines, I'm forced to turn it off. I'm beginning to enjoy the quiet.

Start out with just a few minutes and gradually increase the length of time you zone out. Twenty minutes twice a day has been scientifically proven to improve your health by creating a relaxation response that will even lower high blood pressure. You might enjoy the effects of meditation so much you will want to start a more sophisticated practice. If sitting still is not for you, repetitive exercise can be a moving meditation. Whether you swim, speed walk, run on a treadmill, work out on the elliptical, practice yoga, or dance, clear your mind and feel the energy moving in your body. Nothing is better for being present in the moment. It's time out of time.

I am full of life when I get up in the morning now. I jump out of bed and stretch my arms wide overhead and up to the ceiling to get out the sleeping kinks. I feel good and sexy inhabiting my body. It feels so great to stretch as a cat or dog does after a nap. To set my mood, I think of all the goodness in my life. Reminding myself how much I have to be grateful for is the best way to start my day.

NATURE SAVES ME

My connection to nature is very powerful. It's so easy to take nature for granted—as a background for all the hustle and bustle of life. I find many landscapes nurturing and healing. I rent a single room in Malibu that juts out over the Pacific. My "room with a view" is my weekend getaway. When I'm there, all I can see is sky and ocean. It's magnificent and calming. I love to watch the sun set over the water and hear the cries of the seagulls. I am delighted by an array of God's gifts to man that I see from my room—whales, sea lions, pelicans, and sea turtles, who call the vast Pacific home. I fall asleep to the sound of the sea under my little sanctuary. There are no unwanted distractions or responsibilities. Spending a day or two at my perfect retreat restores me more than being pampered at a spa, though there's nothing wrong with that either. That quiet, uncluttered room in Malibu is my spa.

I always have bird feeders at my places. There is so much activity around a bird feeder. I am mesmerized by watching the pecking order as the birds line up to eat and by listening to their calls and songs. I learned this from my father, who loved looking out the window at the wildlife in our yard. He fed meatballs to rabbits, possums, and gophers. I'd tell him that rabbits don't eat meatballs, but he'd

REAL TIME CHANGE

When I was hungry during the cleanse, I would take a walk or go do errands. Sitting outside in the sunshine was a big help. Getting on the scale was really motivating.

DALE LAWRENCE
DANVERS, MASSACHUSETTS

ME: I never weigh myself—I just go by the way my clothes fit. Nothing like a little sunshine to make you feel good! For me, being outside and moving is a cure-all. I'm a big outside girl!

say, "You watch—they eat Mommy's meatballs." He had names for all the regulars. I remember him standing by the window looking around and asking, "Where's Huxley?" or calling to my mother, "Hurry, Huxley's here, you don't want to miss him." Watching his enjoyment of nature has touched my soul.

One of my favorite occupations is the vegetable garden I plant every summer. No garden gloves for me! I love to feel my hands in the earth and watch things grow and bear fruit. I have a green thumb—my plants just thrive. I think my love of gardening came from my mother's English roots. There is nothing like biting into a tomato, still warm from the sun, which I pick from one of my plants. This year, while doing what I call "extreme gardening," I managed to fracture two fingers as I shoveled and moved a mountain of topsoil. Inside fact: I took off my soft cast when we shot the cover of this book. I just smiled through the pain.

I'm always filled with wonder when I look at a mature oak tree. I think of all the obstacles this old tree had to overcome to grow into a towering presence. Its roots had to grow around rocks. It survived droughts, fierce winds, hurricanes, and freezing weather. Kids climbed it, and swings were hung from its branches. The tree lost limbs over the years, but it kept growing and reaching for the sun. I think of the energy it draws from the sun and the air and how much is required to produce fresh, new leaves in the spring year after year. When I put a log on a crackling fire and warm my hands, I realize that the heat is stored energy from the sun being released as the log burns. It is miraculous to me.

Respecting trees has given me a life lesson. **The fundamental drive in nature is to survive and grow. Since we are part of nature, we are on this earth to do the same, to reach our full possibility, to emerge all of who we are.** Spending time in nature will put your life in perspective in the big scheme of things. You'll see that being bored is a ridiculous waste. You are surrounded by beauty that will elevate you and feed your soul if you stop to notice. I love a tree hugger who has respect for all of life.

In early May, I took a walk with Margaux and her baby girl, Vivienne, in Central Park. We were joined by a woman who lives in Margaux's building. She used to work as a mounted police officer in the park and knows a lot about its history. We strolled through an orchard of Japanese cherry trees in full bloom on the west side of the park. It was magical. Margaux's friend explained that Jackie Onassis had donated a similar grove on the east side. She told us that Jackie moved in nature every day, walking around the reservoir or along the many quiet paths in the park. One of the most iconic women ever, who had been through so much, took comfort from the natural beauty around her. She used her daily exercise as a time to appreciate and revere nature, a perfect restorative for body, mind, and spirit. Jackie Onassis knew what she was doing!

Just about every city and town has a park. Make it a priority to learn about parks and nature preserves where you live, and enjoy them. It will do a lot for your soul.

You deserve to have some quiet time for yourself every day. It can seem a tall order, but it doesn't have to be a lot of time. Schedule this personal time as you would an appointment. You get your chores done and manage to keep your appointments, don't you? Making time for yourself should be a high priority. Worst case scenario: Get up 10 minutes earlier or go to bed 10 minutes later. I take my dog for early morning walks when the world is peaceful and dewy. I love that time of day. A bath before bed can wash away the day's stress. **Your emotional and spiritual health is as important as your physical health. All three are connected and interdependent. You have to take good care of every aspect of yourself to live life to the fullest. I want you to enjoy an elevation of spirit that will expand your focus and make anything seem possible.**

Now that you have made an emotional commitment to get healthy, knowing why revising your diet will get you where you want to be is the best motivation you can have. There is so much confusion about the right way to eat. I know I was baffled by what food and diet fads actually made a difference. When I say that I have eliminated sugar, dairy, and gluten from my diet, many people look at me as if I'm crazy. I'm not, and you'll learn why not in the following pages.

The next chapter gives you the fundamentals of clean eating and explains why eating food close to the source is the best way to go. We have tried to cover it all—processed poison in a box or bag, "frankenfoods" and the threat of GMOs, why sugar is public enemy number one, the truth behind gluten sensitivity, how caffeine and alcohol accelerate aging, why you should eat organic produce and meat, and more. We've tried to give you everything you need to know to motivate you to eat clean permanently.

Nature gives you the face you have at twenty;
it is up to you to merit the face you have at fifty.
—Coco Chanel

Eventually the inner you shapes the outer you.
—Elizabeth Taylor

CHAPTER

4

Navigating the Food Maze

Once you have decided you are worth the effort, you have to take the leap and cut out eating food that is bad for you. Are you ready to make some big changes in your diet? Eating clean will transform you in ways you can't imagine. For me, knowing why I am doing something makes my commitment stronger. **It's easier to resist unhealthy "comfort" food when you know how it hurts you to the point of making you sick.** Before I introduce you to the program, you should have a clear idea of what clean eating is. There is so much noise out there about food it's hard to know what to believe.

Food manufacturers use misleading labels to make you think you're doing the right thing. The more promises in the packaging—100 percent natural, lite, low fat, fat free, low carb, no trans fats, vitamin fortified—the more highly processed the food usually is. By touting the latest buzzwords, food companies are taking advantage of your desire to eat food that is good for you. I understand why so many people get confused, throw up their hands, and go for convenience. When I started, I had no idea how to evaluate which food fad of the moment was actually worth paying attention to. I was lucky to have Lisa Davis to steer me straight. In this chapter, we give you a map to help you find your way through the twists and turns of the current food maze. You will emerge from the confusion with a clear understanding of how to eat in the best possible way for your health and well-being. Your goal is to avoid eating food that is far from the source. Instead, your diet will consist of whole, fresh foods that are alive.

To clean up your act, you have to avoid processed foods, conventionally raised produce and livestock, GMOs (genetically modified organisms), sugar, dairy, gluten—and that includes anything made with flour—caffeine, and alcohol. In the pages that follow, we explain why giving up these foods is essential to maintaining and restoring your health. We examine each item on the elimination list and show its potential to hurt you. If you consider the standard American diet, it's clear that most of us are overdosing on many of these foods, which can create a snowball effect of increasingly severe damage to our bodies.

REAL TIME CHANGE

When I really think about it, I take better care of my car than I do me. I feed it the best gasoline, take it in for oil changes, store it in an indoor garage protecting it from the elements, get it washed regularly, etc. It's time I start filling my tank with the premium gasoline. I'm sure to perform better.

ILIANA GUIBERT
NEW YORK, NEW YORK

ME: I couldn't have said it better myself. Isn't it amazing that so much can be more important to us than paying attention to our health? There is no aging gracefully without good maintenance. So what is it some men call some women—"garage kept"?

Your knee-jerk response to dropping these foods might be like mine was: "No way! That sounds like torture." I guarantee that by the time you finish reading this chapter, you will be seriously motivated to change your eating habits for good because you will know the cost of not paying attention to what you eat. As you begin this introduction to clean eating, keep in mind that you are what you eat. The wrong food choices can make you age faster and are a disaster for your health.

PROCESSED FOOD IS NOT WHOLE

Most foods you eat are processed in some way. In fact, cutting or cooking anything is processing it. That's why they call it a food processor. Vegetables and fruits have to be harvested, ground beef has gone through a machine, and even extra virgin olive oil is the product of pressing. If no chemicals are added, it's still real food. **The processed food that is making people sick all over the world has been chemically processed and made from refined ingredients and artificial substances. Processed foods are so refined they do not resemble the whole foods they come from.**

The packaged foods that you see on the shelves of grocery stores probably have had the life processed out of them. If food is canned, jarred, bagged, or boxed with a long list of ingredients on the label, including many you can't even pronounce, consider it processed. The whole food has been stripped of nutrients during processing, then "enriched" with synthetic vitamins and minerals. Most highly processed foods are full of artificial chemicals that are added to make the food look better and last longer. These additives have many functions. Processed food needs a lot of help. Chemicals are added to stabilize, emulsify, texturize, soften, preserve, sweeten, bleach, color, and hide odors. Many are highly toxic. The Food and Drug Administration has a list of more than 3,000 substances that can be added to foods. Most have never been tested, and some are known to be dangerous.

The highly refined simple carbohydrates found in processed foods are digested quickly. Let me clear something up for you. Not all carbs are created equal. There is a difference between simple and complex carbohydrates. You want to stay away from simple carbs, which are simple sugars. Soda, candy, packaged cereals, jam, fruit juice, and products made from white flour are all

Strategies for Steering Clear of Processed Food

Here are some guidelines for avoiding foods that have nothing to offer you:

Stay out of the center of the grocery store—go for the outside borders. Fresh, unprocessed, whole foods are located on the perimeter, because it is easier to replenish the shelves and bins with fresh food. Produce, meat, seafood, eggs, and dairy are almost always located along the walls. Packaged foods are filled with stabilizers and preservatives to have a long shelf life. The exception is that most supermarkets today have an aisle and freezer section of healthy processed foods, usually called "organic." The number of gluten-free products is growing.

Be very selective about what you buy in bags, cans, and boxes. Most packaged foods have been processed and enriched with salt, sweetener, fat, and other additives to compensate for the flavor and nutrition lost during the refining and processing. It's imperative to read the ingredients list. I'm happy to say that many companies are responding to the growing demand for healthy food. Most grocery stores have special sections offering healthy options.

Be careful if a label has more than five ingredients. The more ingredients a product has, the more it has been processed. The food is man-made and far removed from nature. For a more detailed explanation of how to read a label, see page 156.

If any of the first three ingredients ends in "ose," do not put it in your basket. "Ose" means sugar. Many of the sugars used by the food industry are high in calories and bad for you. Sugar is added back into food, because the food is so highly processed it loses its flavor.

Avoid white food. White bread, white rice, and white pasta are made from bleached and enriched wheat flour or grain. When grains are refined, the bran and germ, the most nutritious parts of the grain, are removed. The starches from refined grains feed sugar addictions, because they break down to sugar so quickly. The flour or grain is bleached, which strips it of all the fiber and nutrients. The manufacturer then adds fiber and vitamins, which your body does not absorb, because they do not occur in nature. When it comes to potatoes—America's favorite vegetable—they break down to sugar very quickly in your body and set off the blood sugar roller coaster.

simple carbs. Eating simple carbs leads to spikes in blood sugar and insulin levels. This can lead to carb cravings later when blood sugar levels plummet. Complex carbohydrates, including vegetables and beans, are known as starches. They contain fiber, vitamins, and minerals and are digested slowly, making you feel full longer. The Clean Up Your Act Diet is heavy on complex carbs.

Processed foods are quickly digested, because most of the fiber has been removed. Fiber slows down the absorption of carbohydrates and fills you up with fewer calories. Though processed food tends to be much more caloric than whole food, you only burn half as many calories digesting and metabolizing it.

"Big Food" loads their products with hidden sugar, sodium, and fat, because our tastebuds and appetite respond to sweet, salty, and fatty foods. Food manufacturers are engineering their products to stimulate the reward center of the brain. We have become high-flavor addicts, and sugar is the drug of choice. Just as with any addiction, we need to consume more and more to be satisfied. **Junk food is designed to hijack the biochemistry of your brain and keep you hungry all the time so that you buy more.** The maneuver is comparable to the way the tobacco industry doctored cigarettes to hook users before the industry was regulated. It's like a bartender who lays out salty treats so that you drink more.

REAL TIME CHANGE

I liked that the cleanse was not about weight loss but about cleaning up my act. I know how to eat well and I do. Historically, I binged on sugar and salty snacks, and previously kept myself stimulated with caffeine. I needed to end my own cycle.

Now that I am eating clean, my energy is steady all day. I wake up feeling ready to take on my day. My head is clear, my body feels great as I crave fruit, nuts, and meat—no more Doritos bingeing, no more sugar-loaded snacks as attempted pick-me-ups.

MICHELE BLOOM
SOUTH ORANGE, NEW JERSEY

ME: Eating clean does even you out—no more edginess and no crashes. Without the chemically induced extremes, your energy flows naturally when you clean up your act. You are craving things that will actually nourish you.

It's so wrong! They don't even care that they are destroying our health. They just want to make more money. It's infuriating.

Processed food is often high in unhealthy fats like trans fats, processed vegetable oils, and cheap fats like soybean oil. The fats used in most processed food contain excessive amounts of omega-6 fatty acids, which can cause inflammation in the body. Inflammation is the first step on the road to disease.

Trading convenience for your health is not worth it. **You will find that when you start to eat clean, your tastebuds will respond to simple flavors in their natural state. The tastes are subtle compared to the synthetic flavor overload of processed foods.** After 4 years of eating clean, processed food tastes disgusting to me. It has totally lost its appeal. Recently, I tried a piece of licorice, which I used to eat by the bagful. It tasted so terrible that I had to spit it out! It's great to open my kitchen cabinets now and find only a handful of healthy staples, such as quinoa, a jar of almond butter, and cans of organic beans. No more junk in my house!

THE WORST INGREDIENT IN THE MODERN DIET

Though sugar is the body's fuel of choice, we eat way too much of it. Sugar found in fruits and vegetables is perfectly healthy. The sugar added to food during processing is the problem. The American Heart Association recommends that women get no more than 24 grams of added sugar a day. That's about 6 teaspoons or 100 calories. A 12-ounce can of regular soda contains 9 teaspoons of sugar, more than the recommended amount of sugar for an entire day. Just one can of soda a day could lead to 15 pounds of weight gain in a single year. Today, the average American woman has about 18 teaspoons of sugar every day, three times what is recommended. **On average, Americans consume 156 pounds of sugar a year. Believe it or not, that's 3 pounds or 6 cups of sugar a week. No one is spooning out that much sugar. Most of it is hidden in processed food.** Sugar is found in everything from crackers to salad dressing. But sodas, energy drinks, and sports drinks are by far the biggest sources of sugar in the average diet, accounting for more than one-third the added sugar consumed in this country. Cakes, cookies, pastries, ice cream, frozen yogurt, candy, and breakfast cereals are the other major culprits.

Sugar Decoded

Food manufacturers very cleverly disguise the presence of sugar in their products by using different names. Sometimes they use small amounts of several different sugars so that none of them appears in the top ingredients. Labels can make sugar sound like a healthier ingredient, such as "organic dehydrated cane juice." That doesn't sound so bad, does it? Fruit juice concentrates, which sound all right, are used sometimes, but when fruit juice is concentrated, guess what you get? Sugar! The following list is not close to complete but gives you an idea of how far Big Food will go to cover up the presence of sugar in processed food.

- Agave nectar
- Barley malt syrup
- Beet sugar
- Brown rice syrup
- Brown sugar
- Buttered syrup
- Cane crystals (or, even better, cane juice crystals)
- Cane juice solids
- Cane sugar
- Caramel
- Carob syrup
- Coconut sugar, or coconut palm sugar
- Corn sweetener
- Corn syrup, or corn syrup solids
- Date sugar
- Dehydrated cane juice
- Dextrin
- Dextrose
- Diastase
- Diastatic malt
- Evaporated cane juice
- Fructose
- Fruit juice concentrate or crystals
- Glucose
- Golden syrup
- High-fructose corn syrup
- Honey
- Invert sugar
- Lactose
- Maltodextrin
- Maltose
- Malt syrup
- Maple syrup
- Molasses
- Palm sugar
- Raw sugar
- Refiner's syrup
- Rice syrup
- Saccharose
- Sorghum or sorghum syrup
- Sucrose
- Syrup
- Treacle
- Turbinado sugar
- Xylose
- Yellow sugar

All of these are just plain sugar to your body.

Glucose and Fructose

To understand why eating too much sucrose, as sugar is called, is dangerous to your health, you have to know what it is composed of. Before sugar enters the digestive track, it is broken down into two simple sugars: glucose and fructose.

Glucose is also called blood sugar. Your body breaks down carbohydrates to glucose and uses that form of sugar for energy. Glucose is stored in muscle cells to provide energy when it is needed. Glucose is also stored in the liver as glycogen for later energy use. Elevated levels of blood sugar cause insulin to be secreted. Insulin helps glucose enter cells.

The body uses fructose differently. It is not used as an energy source for muscles or the brain. While just about every cell can break down glucose for energy, liver cells are the only ones that can handle fructose. If there is too much fructose in your diet, the liver creates fat, which accumulates in liver cells. The buildup results in nonalcoholic fatty liver disease, and the last thing you want is a sick liver. Too much fructose:

- Increases harmful LDL
- Elevates triglycerides
- Promotes buildup of visceral fat around the organs that is hard to lose
- Increases blood pressure
- Leads to insulin resistance, a precursor to diabetes
- Increases free radicals that can damage DNA and cells

REAL TIME CHANGE

Three weeks without Coke? After going through initial withdrawal symptoms, I feel great and really don't miss it. The fact that I had to go through withdrawal from soda really scared me, and now I don't want any part of chemicals anymore!

STEPHANIE AUGELLO
BETHLEHEM, PENNSYLVANIA

ME: Caffeine and sugar—a killer combination! If you had a sip of cola now, you would not believe how bad it tastes. You won't know what you liked about it before.

All of these changes are bad for your heart and arteries as well.

Fructose is found naturally in many fruits and vegetables and added to beverages like soda. Fructose used as an additive is not good for you. You don't want your liver to overwork metabolizing fructose. You want your liver to be able to eliminate toxins from your body. Eating clean will do that for you. Avoid high fructose corn syrup—a major ingredient in sodas—like the plague!

Public Enemy #1

I'm not criminalizing sugar without cause. If I do only one thing in this chapter, I want to convince you that consuming too much sugar is one of the worst things you can do. That sweet tooth of yours can destroy your health. Sugar is high on my hit list, because eating too much is so damaging. If you're breathing, you have to be aware of some of sugar's bad effects, but I'd bet there are others you don't even suspect. Here are some of the awful things too much sugar can do to your health:

Sugar causes cavities. You've known this since you were a child. Tooth decay happens when the bacteria that line the teeth feed on simple sugars, creating acid that destroys enamel. Sour candies are particularly treacherous.

Sugar has no essential nutrients. Sugar's high count of "empty" calories is pure energy. No protein, fiber, essential fats, vitamins, or minerals are found in sugar. If you are eating a lot of sugar, you're probably skipping things you should be eating instead. The result: nutritional deficiencies. And, of course, you know what happens to that excess sugar.

Sugar in excess will cause you to gain weight. Okay, this is obvious. You pack on the pounds, because the energy sugar provides is stored if you don't use it. Don't fool yourself. It takes a lot of intense exercise to burn sufficient calories to avoid weight gain. From my point of view, cutting back on sugar is so much easier.

Sugar accelerates aging. Eating too much sugar intensifies glycation, a principal process of internal aging that breaks down collagen. Collagen keeps your skin supple and resilient. When this protein breaks down, your skin loses volume and begins to sag and wrinkle.

Sugar will turn off your appetite control. Eating too much sugar reduces the effectiveness of the hormone leptin, which controls appetite. When your body doesn't respond to the leptin produced by your fat cells, your brain never receives the "I'm full" message. You are always hungry, and you gain weight and inches, because the fructose is stored in fat cells.

Too much sugar will raise your blood pressure. Hypertension is usually associated with salty foods, but eating lots of added sugar has been connected to high blood pressure as well. Consuming ⅓ cup or 5 tablespoons or more of sugar each day has been strongly associated with an elevated risk of high blood pressure.

Too many high-sugar meals will eventually make your body resistant to insulin, the first step to developing type 2 diabetes, metabolic syndrome, and cancer. The excess sugar in your bloodstream increases your body's demand for insulin, which converts food to usable energy. If your insulin levels are consistently high, you reduce your body's sensitivity to the hormone and blood sugar levels build up. Symptoms include fatigue, hunger, brain fog, high blood pressure, and extra weight around the middle. Insulin resistance is usually not diagnosed until it develops into full-blown type 2 diabetes. People who drink sugar-sweetened beverages have up to an 83 percent higher risk of type 2 diabetes. If that's not enough to make you want to change your ways, an increased level of insulin in the bloodstream may also act as growth factors for cancer.

Too much sugar can overload your liver. When fructose accumulates in the liver, it can cause a stress response. Your liver goes into overdrive, which exacerbates inflammation. Eventually, you can develop nonalcoholic fatty liver disease.

Sugar raises your bad cholesterol and promotes heart disease. Evidence is mounting that fructose may be one of the leading drivers of heart disease. Large amounts of fructose can raise triglycerides, LDL cholesterol (which I call "lousy cholesterol" to remember it's the bad one), blood sugar, and insulin levels, and increase abdominal obesity in as little as 10 weeks. These are all major risk factors for heart disease. When I learned this, I thought, "How long have I been eating bags of candy? A lot longer than 10 weeks!" I had to drop sugar from my diet before I did some serious damage to myself.

I hope this list is enough to make you gun-shy about sugar, as it did for me. You'll feel so much better when you drop it from your diet.

Artificial Sweeteners Are Not the Answer

Though artificial sweeteners contain no calories, they can contribute to weight problems and make you fat. Your body judges the number of calories in what you eat by how it tastes. Sugar substitutes separate the taste of sweetness from the calories. When you drink a diet soda, your tastebuds communicate to your brain that energy is coming in, but your body does not get the fuel it expects. More signals are sent to your brain that the body needs to be fed. Artificial sweeteners can upset your food chemistry and interfere with your body's natural regulating processes. In other words, artificial sweeteners make you hungry.

They trick your body in another way. Artificial sweeteners are 200 to 13,000 times as sweet as sugar. The "feel-good" hormones in your brain, called endorphins, respond to this extremely strong signal. As more endorphins are produced, your pleasure increases, which leads you to eat more. That's what's known as a sugar high. The taste of sweetness is addictive. The more sweets you eat, the more you need to feel satisfied.

A friend once observed, "Thin people don't drink diet cola." Gaining weight has to do with more than calories!

"FRANKENFOODS"—BEYOND PROCESSING

I kept hearing about GMOs and the controversy around whether they are safe or not. I had no idea what people were talking about, but it seemed important to find out what was happening to our food supply. I knew that GMOs had been banned in Europe but not in the United States. It made me nervous. It's not that I'm against progress—I'm just suspicious about trying to improve on nature. What I discovered confirmed that there was reason to be cautious.

Genetic engineers have been experimenting with our food supply since the 1990s. They are creating genetically modified organisms (GMOs) by moving genes from one organism to another. They extract specific genes from the DNA of an organism and splice those genes into the DNA of another. The genes that are transferred can come from viruses, bacteria, insects, animals, and even humans. These experimental combinations of genes from different species create unstable cellular structures that do not occur in nature or in traditional crossbreeding.

This technique is used on crop plants grown to be eaten by animals and humans. The plants are modified to enhance desired traits. Genetic engineering can create plants with exactly the desired characteristics very quickly. Some of the qualities the biotech companies are working on include higher crop yields, pest resistance, herbicide tolerance so that weeds can be killed chemically without hurting the crop, disease resistance, cold and drought tolerance, and nutritional and flavor enrichment.

Genetically modified crops have been banned as food ingredients in Europe and elsewhere. China, Russia, and about 60 other countries require labeling if a food contains GMO ingredients. Here in the United States, government supervision is very lax. The Food and Drug Administration (FDA) has neither banned GMOs from the food supply nor required labeling. Without labeling, there is no way to know which foods contain GMOs. Did you get that? Even China requires labeling, but we don't here in the United States. We don't even get to make informed choices. One thing is certain: genetically modified organisms cannot be used in any stage of organic farming. When you read about the dangers associated with GMOs, you will have even more reason to eat fresh, organic food.

Since GMOs have not been tested for long-term health impacts, the jury is still out on whether they are unhealthy. They simply haven't been in the food supply long enough to know their effects on us. Animal studies of the effects of GMOs have been done that show organ damage, digestive and immune system disorders, accelerated aging, and infertility.

However, the National Institutes of Health reported on a study that found toxic insecticide produced by genetically modified corn in the blood of pregnant women and their unborn babies. That is enough for me! And it gets worse. Since GMOs were introduced, the percentage of Americans with three or more chronic illnesses has jumped from 7 to 13 percent in 9 years. Food allergies have skyrocketed. Genetic engineering can expose humans to toxins and allergens that have never been seen before. No one knows how GMOs interact.

There are so many unanswered questions. At this point, **there is not sufficient research to confirm whether GMOs are a contributing factor to the rise in allergies and disease, but the American Academy of Environmental Medicine advises us not to wait before we start to protect our children and**

ourselves. I'm not willing to wait for proof. How long did it take the FDA to decide that cigarette smoking is bad for your health? How many people got sick and died because they smoked? My father was among them. I won't take a chance on my health.

Plants genetically engineered to resist herbicides have increased the amount of herbicide used. Overuse of Roundup produced "superweeds" resistant to the herbicide. Farmers are using even more toxic herbicides every year, which hurts the environment and invades our food. The same thing happens with pesticides. Foods are being altered to minimize the need for pesticides by making pesticides part of the plant. Genetically engineered crops manufacture their own pesticides, which increases the pesticide contamination in our food and land. In time, insects will become resistant to pesticides, which just goes to show you that you can't outsmart nature.

What worries me is that there is no way to control the spread of GMOs. Once GMOs are dispersed in the environment, it is impossible to control them. Wind, birds, and insects can carry genetically altered seeds into nearby fields and farther. Pollen from genetically modified plants can cross-pollinate with natural crops. GMO pollution has the potential to threaten our food supply and the health of future generations. GM crops can harm birds, insects, amphibians, marine ecosystems, and soil organisms. No wonder they're called frankenfoods!

Genetically modified seeds first appeared in the food supply in 1990s. Today, about 30,000 genetically modified food products sit on grocery store shelves in the United States, none with a label. **GMOs are now used in as much as 80 percent of conventional processed food—another reason to eat whole, fresh food.** Green America compiled a list of the GMO ingredients to avoid. The percentage represents how much of that US crop has been genetically modified.

- **Soybean:** 94 percent in 2011. Used in nonorganic soy products such as tofu, soy milk, soy sauce, miso, and tempeh, and the emulsifier lecithin. This is why you have to avoid soy products on the Clean Up Your Act Diet.
- **Corn:** 88 percent in 2011. GM corn is found in hundreds of products, including breakfast cereals, corn flour products like tortillas and

chips, corn oil products like mayonnaise, and anything sweetened with high fructose corn syrup. (Michael Pollan, in his book *The Omnivore's Dilemma*, described North Americans as "corn chips with legs"!)

- **Cottonseed:** 90 percent in 2011. The oil is an ingredient in margarine, salad dressings, and frying oil for potato chips and other snacks. None of these foods is on your "to eat" list.
- **Canola oil:** 90 percent in 2010. Popular cooking oil. Olive oil and grapeseed oil are better choices.
- **US-grown papaya:** 80 percent in 2010. Hawaiian papaya was genetically engineered in the late 1990s, and GMOs were introduced to Florida plantations in 2009.
- **Sugar beets:** 95 percent in 2005. About half the sugar produced in the United States is made from sugar beets. Something else not to like about sugar!
- **Milk:** 17 percent in 2007. A GM growth hormone is injected into dairy cows to boost milk production. Not only are those cows shot up with a growth hormone, but it's genetically modified—a double whammy.
- **Aspartame:** 100 percent in 1965. Aspartame, an artificial sweetener, is derived from GM microorganisms. It is found in more than 6,000 products, including diet sodas. Forget about artificial sweeteners. You don't need those chemicals.

REAL TIME CHANGE

This is much easier than I was anticipating—simple and satisfying. Just went shopping all organic. Going to keep truckin'. It's never too late to start feeling better.

JEANIE CIUPPA SANTACROCE
LODI, NEW JERSEY

ME: It is easy, and you've just started to feel better. I promise in a couple more weeks you will be elated.

Since GMO ingredients are found in the great majority of processed foods, the only way to avoid them is to eat whole, clean, and organic foods.

WHY EAT ORGANIC PRODUCE?

We ask you to eat organic fruits and vegetables during the cleanse and highly recommend making the switch to organic produce permanent. It's like organizing your closets. After you have sorted through your clothes and shoes and gotten rid of things you don't wear, and your closets look like a high-end, minimal boutique, you wouldn't rehang the discarded clothes. You want to keep your closets and drawers in a pristine state. **Once you have cleansed, you'll want to avoid eating toxic foods. Why mess up what you have worked so hard to achieve?**

First, let's clear up any labeling confusion. "Natural" and "organic" are not interchangeable. Many food labels read "all natural," "free-range," or "hormone free," but do not assume they are organic. Only foods that are grown and processed according to USDA organic standards can be labeled organic. Organic food differs from conventionally produced food in the way it is grown, handled, and processed.

I prefer organic produce and meat, because they taste better. One of the reasons organic food is more flavorful is that the plants and animals are allowed to mature naturally. Aside from tasting better, there are a number of reasons eating organic is the way to go.

Here's a little test you can do. Take a knife and scrape the skin of a conventionally raised apple. I was shocked by how much wax I was able to scrape off. It's unbelievable how much wax is used to keep the apples moist and fresh longer. Conventional farming practices are insidious. Organic apples may not shine like apples not raised organically, but no one is "improving" their very nutritious skin.

The chart on page 48 compares conventional and organic farming methods.

Organic food is usually 20 percent more expensive than chemically grown food, because production and postharvest handling costs are higher. In weighing the price difference, you have to consider the cost of the potential health damage to you, your family, and the planet when you choose to eat conventionally farmed food. The answer is clear to me.

CONVENTIONAL FARMING	ORGANIC FARMING
Uses chemical fertilizers that affect the soil and water supply.	Uses natural fertilizers such as manure and compost that feed soil and build soil matter.
More than 400 chemical pesticides are routinely used to protect crops from molds, insects, and disease. They are designed to be toxic. Residues remain on food even after washing. The pesticides are endocrine disruptors. They linger in your body and remain long after eating. They have been linked to cancer and asthma. These toxins run off into the soil and water supply.	Uses natural pesticides, bugs and birds, mating disruption, traps and barriers, careful crop selection, and beneficial microorganisms to control crop-damaging pests.
Synthetic herbicides are used to kill weeds. The toxins enter the soil and eventually run off to the water supply.	Uses crop rotation, mulching, mechanical tillage and hand weeding, cover crops to manage weed growth.
Can use preservatives, waxing, artificial sweeteners, colorings, flavorings, and MSG.	Does not use food additives, processing aids, or fortifying agents. Does not wax produce to preserve.
Robs food of more than 60 natural and trace elements. Poisons our food supply, the air we breathe, the water we drink, and the soil in which crops are grown.	Some claim organic food is an average of 25 percent more nutritious with higher levels of beta-carotene, antioxidants, flavonoids, essential fatty acids, and vitamins C, D, and E. (These findings are controversial, because of measurement problems in the studies.) Organic farming practices are designed to benefit the environment by reducing pollution and conserving water and soil quality.
Uses genetically modified seeds.	No genetically modified material used in farming.

THE CARE AND FEEDING OF LIVESTOCK

For the cleanse, you will only be eating chicken and beef that are organic. As you would expect, conventional and organic methods for raising livestock are radically different. Unlike conventionally raised livestock, organic livestock must be kept in living conditions that accommodate the natural behavior of the animals. Conventional meat and poultry are manufactured in feedlots. The facilities are like factories that house tens of thousands of animals in deplorable conditions. They are crowded in so close together that they can hardly move. It's like living your entire life on a subway car at the peak of rush hour. Normal behavior is impossible. At some factory farms, animals do not even have space to lie down.

Disease can spread quickly under these conditions. The animals are dosed with antibiotics to keep them from getting sick. I was shocked to learn that half the antibiotics used in the world are given to animals at feedlots. In contrast, most organically raised livestock have access to pastures in the open air and are free to move. Since organic regulations do not allow medical treatments unless the animal is sick, livestock are not given antibiotics as a preventive measure. Instead, livestock diseases and parasites are controlled through nonmedical preventive measures such as rotational grazing, balanced diet, sanitary housing, and stress reduction. Scientists are concerned that the use of antibiotics on feedlots could lead to "superbugs," strains of bacteria that resist antibiotics and can be passed to humans. Hello, avian flu!

Cattle are meant to eat grass. Their digestive system is designed for it. Organic livestock must be fed a diet of organic agricultural products, grass, and grains that have not been sprayed with toxins. **Look for grass-fed, organic beef when you are at the market. Conventionally raised cattle eat soybeans and corn that have been produced with many toxins and GMOs. The toxins are stored in the fat cells of cattle.** Cattle do not graze at a feedlot. There is no grass, and they cannot move. Cattle that are fed grains alone have more deadly *E. coli* bacteria in their intestines and feces, which can contaminate meat during slaughter.

At feedlots, livestock are treated with growth and other hormones and supplements so that they grow faster and can be slaughtered sooner to save the cost of letting animals develop and grow naturally. When you eat the meat, you absorb those hormones and antibiotics. Organically raised livestock is not treated with hormones or antibiotics to fatten them up for slaughter.

Feedlots hurt the environment. They produce millions of tons of manure that contaminate water supplies. Sometimes conventional farmers collect manure and spray it on the land. The fertilizers, pesticides, and antibiotics present in the waste material can create health problems for people in the area. The *E. coli* in the manure can contaminate vegetable crops. In organic pastures, where the grass is not treated with synthetic fertilizers or pesticides, manure from the animals is used instead, a practical way to dispose of waste.

When I was working for Riverkeeper with Robert F. Kennedy Jr., we visited the Black Warrior River in Birmingham, Alabama. The runoff from the local pig farms had destroyed the river. It was filled with trash. You couldn't fish it anymore. Nothing could possibly live in that river. We own our waterways. We have to protect them. We can't allow them to become horribly polluted. We have to keep our water clean. One way to help is to buy organic.

Aside from animal rights issues, which are significant, there are many convincing reasons to choose organic poultry and beef over conventionally raised livestock. Your goal is to reduce your exposure to harmful substances. When you eat organic meat, you are protecting yourself and the environment.

Some time ago, I read a book on anger by a Vietnamese Zen monk named Thich Nhat Hanh. I remember to this day what he said about fear and anger in livestock. I want to quote him from a speech he gave, because his compassionate understanding is so remarkable. I left the words as he spoke them:

> The way we grow our food, the way we raise our stock, our cattle to eat might be very violent. We destroy a lot of forest land. We pollute a lot of the water just by making meat, and the meat we eat may contain a lot of anger and violence. . . . Imagine a chicken that is raised in a cage like this. In modern chicken farms, each chicken has only one space . . . like a box and in the whole life of chicken, where the chicken has to live, another lay eggs and finally to be killed for the meat. The chickens are so angry that, if there's a chance, it will attack the next chicken with its beak and that's why they practice this cutting off the point of the beak of chicken. Imagine you eat a piece of chicken like that. Every cell of the chicken contains anger and despair.

How do we raise our calf cows? When the calf is born from the cow, they take it away from the cow, and the calf never know the joy of drinking the milk from its mother. They raise the calf in a space like this. The calf cannot run and play like in the old time. It has to stay in just one place. One hundred days later, it will be killed for meat. . . . We are ruining our planet by the way of eating. We are bringing a lot of toxins into our body and into the body of our family, and that is why practice in mindful eating is very important.

When you eat chicken and beef that have been raised conventionally, you are also consuming emotional toxins—the fear and anger these animals experience all their lives. That should make you think twice when you buy meat.

REAL TIME CHANGE

I would recommend to anyone to see how they feel without gluten, sugar, or dairy. It is truly amazing!

AMY MURPHY
NEW YORK, NEW YORK

ME: It's true. You'll be shocked at how much better you feel. Our bodies react quickly. No one believes it until trying it out. It seems like major deprivation, but it's not.

GLUTEN FREE

You can't walk through a market without a "gluten-free" label jumping out at you from all sorts of products. If you're like I was, I had no idea what gluten was or why I should avoid it. I want to clear it up for you. The latest dietary craze is gluten free. Gluten is a protein found in some grains. About 1 percent of the population is so sensitive to gluten that even a small amount can make them extremely sick. The condition is known as celiac disease. If you have celiac disease, gluten damages the lining of the small intestine, which develops into a wide range of health problems that include chronic diarrhea and abdominal cramping.

In the past 50 years, our consumption of gluten has increased significantly, thanks to all the processed foods in our diet made with highly refined wheat flour. This highly refined flour triggers sugar addiction, because it is quickly digested. The surge in sugar in the bloodstream stimulates the pleasure centers in your brain, which leads to needing more sugar to feel good. Here is a helpful tip: **If you eat gluten free, it is easier to reduce your sugar habit.**

Our gluten overload has produced a condition known as gluten sensitivity that affects millions of people. Latest estimates are that 6 percent of people in the United States—as many as 18 million—suffer the symptoms of gluten sensitivity. When gluten-sensitive people consume the protein, they experience stomach pains, heartburn, bloating, rashes, headache, joint pains, fatigue, insomnia, and brain fog. Sounds like the story of my life before I started to eat gluten free! It's worth swearing off gluten just to see if some of your aging and stress symptoms disappear as mine did. Some people experience no signs or symptoms after eating gluten, but being symptom free may not reflect the damage that is being done to their small intestines.

You should avoid food and drinks that contain:

- Wheat
- Barley
- Rye
- Oats (unless certified gluten free)
- Malt (a derivative of barley used in malt flavoring and malt vinegar)
- Brewer's yeast
- Triticale (a cross between wheat and rye)

Certain grains, such as oats, can be contaminated with wheat during the growing and processing stages. If you love your oatmeal, look for the gluten-free label.

Wheat and Gluten in Camo

Avoiding wheat can be tricky, because wheat goes by a number of names. I am a food detective when it comes to reading ingredients lists. If I find any gluten-containing grains, back it goes on the shelf. Wheat-derivative products to look for include:

- Bulgur
- Durum flour
- Einkorn
- Emmer
- Farina
- Farro
- Graham flour
- Kamut
- Semolina
- Spelt

I'm sure you're not surprised to hear that gluten hides in many prepared foods. Unless they're labeled gluten free, you should avoid or carefully study the labels of:

- Beer
- Bran
- Candies
- Cereals
- Couscous
- French fries
- Gravies
- Imitation meat or seafood
- Processed luncheon meats
- Ramen
- Salad dressings
- Sauces, including soy sauce
- Seasoned rice mixes
- Seasoned snack foods, such as potato and tortilla chips
- Self-basting poultry
- Some medications and vitamins, which may use gluten as a binding agent
- Soups and soup bases

- Udon
- Vegetables in sauce

Since gluten sensitivity is on the rise, food manufacturers are developing an increasing number of gluten-free products. **Buyer beware: Gluten-free packaged products are often just as high in saturated fat, sugar, and salt as other junk food. These products sometimes use refined ingredients like white rice flour or fillers like potato starch that can raise your blood sugar and trigger cravings.** Read the labels of gluten-free products carefully. And a friendly reminder: Just because cookies are gluten free doesn't mean you can eat the whole box! I'm not proud of it, but it's happened to me. I've learned to dole out the portion size and put away the box before snacking.

REAL TIME CHANGE

Having eliminated dairy and gluten from my diet, my knees are pain free. That alone is a good enough reason to remain off of dairy and gluten. Before I started the cleanse, I was noticing that by the end of the day, my ankles would get very swollen. Now, no more swelling!

MICHELE BLOOM
SOUTH ORANGE, NEW JERSEY

ME: This was huge for me. That's exactly what I experienced. My aches and pains disappeared. Many of us have sensitivities to foods we are completely unaware of until we stop eating them.

MILK MYTHS

Milk and dairy products are not as healthy as you've always been told. **Humans are the only species that continues to drink milk after infancy, and the milk of a different species at that. The fact is that the majority of us naturally stop producing enough lactase—the enzyme needed to metabolize lactose, the sugar in milk—sometime between the ages of 2 and 5.** Approximately 75 percent of the world's population is genetically unable to digest lactose properly. The problem, called lactose intolerance, can lead to bloating, gas, abdominal pain, constipation, and diarrhea and can aggravate irritable bowel syndrome.

Most people are not even aware of their intolerance until they eliminate dairy for a few weeks and start feeling better.

Casein and whey, proteins found in milk, can also cause an allergic reaction. A casein allergy occurs when the immune system mistakenly thinks the protein is harmful and produces allergic antibodies for protection. The symptoms are similar to any allergy: swelling of the lips, mouth, tongue, face, or throat; skin reactions; itchy eyes; nasal congestion; sneezing; coughing; or wheezing. The symptoms can be severe. A reaction to casein can be misinterpreted as a sensitivity to other substances.

Despite the powerful ad campaigns, dairy products are just not that good for you. If you don't drink raw, organic milk, you are dealing with the same issues as you would if you ate traditionally raised beef. Milk is highly processed by the time you pour it into a glass. The hormones that are naturally present in cow's milk are stronger than human hormones. **The steroids and hormones the cows are given to plump them up and increase milk production can affect your hormone balance.** Normally, cows do not produce milk for more than 6 months a year. When they are treated with hormones, they produce milk 10 months a year. Commercial feed for cows contains a list of ingredients you want to avoid like the plague: genetically modified corn, genetically modified soy, animal products, chicken manure, cottonseed, pesticides, and antibiotics. Pesticides, hormones, and antibiotics find their way into the milk and dairy products we consume.

And let's not forget that cows do not roam free, grazing on pastures of green grass. Dairy cows live in confined, inhumane conditions. I have to believe that the misery of their lives affects their milk in ways we don't know—just like the meat and poultry that come from feedlots.

Now for the processing part of the equation. Most dairy products are pasteurized to kill potentially harmful bacteria. During the process, vitamins, proteins, and enzymes are destroyed. Enzymes aid digestion. When pasteurization destroys them, milk is more difficult to digest, which strains our own enzyme system. Most milk is also homogenized. When raw milk sits, the fat separates from the rest of the liquid and rises to the top, forming a layer of cream. I remember old milk bottles with a bulb on top so that the heavy cream rose to the top; this was in the days before almost all milk was homogenized. The process of homogenizing keeps the fat molecules dispersed throughout the milk, so that the separation does not occur. Homogenization uses high pressure to force the milk through very small tubes, which causes the fat globules to break down into smaller particles. This process takes milk even further from its natural state.

When metabolized, dairy products are acid forming. You don't want your body to become more acidic. When our bodies get out of balance, acid-balancing mechanisms come into play. Calcium, which is alkaline, is stored in the bones. The bones release calcium to combat the acidity. Over time, bones can become fragile. **We are told to drink milk to build strong bones, when the opposite is true. Countries in Africa and Asia with the lowest rates of dairy and calcium consumption have the lowest rates of osteoporosis.**

REAL TIME CHANGE

My skin looks so vibrant! It looks better than it has in a long time. Although I do not have full-blown arthritis, I work with my hands a lot— either on the computer or sewing, knitting, crafts. My wrists used to bother me after extensive use. They have not bothered me in weeks. Some say that it is due to eliminating dairy.

LORETTA LANG STOKES
BEVERLY, MASSACHUSETTS

ME: Changing the way you eat and giving your liver a deep cleanse has had positive results in just 6 weeks. Keep up the good work. You will continue to feel better.

Dairy products are mucous-forming and can intensify seasonal allergies, postnasal drip, sinus problems, and ear infections. Research has linked dairy with arthritis and joint pain. And there may be a link between dairy products and cancer. The American Cancer Society says that dairy consumption increases the level of insulin-like growth factor (IGF-1), a known promoter of cancer.

You will not be eating dairy products during your 2-week cleanse. You'll be surprised at how good you feel. It made a big difference for me. Now I allow myself a little milk in my coffee, if rice or almond milk is not available, but I'm just about dairy free and wouldn't think of going back. When something is working, why change it?

REAL TIME CHANGE

This plan was definitely a bit daunting for me—no sugar, alcohol, dairy, or bread? I lived on those! I knew it was well balanced and would change my eating habits for the better. I didn't see it as a short-term diet, but more of a change in lifestyle, which is something I desperately needed.

ELIZABETH BLOOM
NEW YORK, NEW YORK

ME: We all lived on those things. You are not alone. I wanted to explain why you are eliminating sugar, dairy, gluten, caffeine, and alcohol from your diet in this chapter. If you understand how these foods are aging you, giving them up becomes a no-brainer. I had Lisa to answer all of my questions during my transition to eating clean, and I had a ton of them. We're asking you to make radical changes in your eating habits. It's important for you to know why so that you own this program.

THE #1 PSYCHOACTIVE DRUG IN THE WORLD

I like a good cup of coffee to get me going in the morning. I love the ritual of making coffee to start the day. It smells so good. I needed that energy charge several times a day to wake me up, keep my energy high, and improve my focus when I was lagging.

When Lisa made me aware of how hazardous too much coffee could be for my health, I was determined to cut back on my coffee habit. Decaf wasn't the answer, because it is so highly processed. I managed to substitute herbal teas and hot lemon water during the cleanse and for a long time after. I'm now officially addicted to licorice mint tea, which beats candy. Once I got my energy back, I didn't need to depend on coffee as a stimulant. To be honest, reducing my coffee intake was challenging for me. I had withdrawal symptoms—headache, fatigue, and jumpiness. After a few days, I was better than ever. Four years after I began working on my transformation, I have been able to keep my coffee consumption to a cup or two a day, which is within the safe zone. Even so, it would be better if I abstained from coffee completely. As I said, I'm a work in progress!

Caffeine is the most widely used psychoactive drug in the world, and it's unregulated. A psychoactive substance is one that has an effect on the brain. The Food and Drug Administration says that at least 80 percent of adults in the West consume caffeine in amounts large enough to affect their brains. Caffeine has been so incorporated into our diets that we have stopped considering it potentially harmful to our health. Coffee and tea are natural sources of caffeine. **Higher-dosed caffeinated products like colas, sports and energy drinks, weight loss and energy pills, and even pain relievers have slipped into our diets. It is easy to overdose without realizing it.** Pay attention to how much caffeine you are getting from food and beverages. It may be more than you think. Your estimate might be a little low, because not all foods and drinks list caffeine. For example, chocolate contains a small amount of caffeine but doesn't list it on the label.

REAL TIME CHANGE

I craved coffee and black tea in the worst way throughout the 2 weeks. There were so many triggers—the smell, the sight of a travel mug, parties— but my normal routine was the largest trigger. I never admitted I had a caffeine issue, but clearly I had a large one. I had gotten in the habit of skipping breakfast and having one cup of coffee. That one cup turned into two and sometimes three several days a week. Each afternoon and after dinner I had black tea and will admit I would drink another cup at certain times in the day to chase away hunger. All this was done under the banner of avoiding calories. How misguided.

DIANE ARPINO
RAMSEY, NEW JERSEY

ME: One of my good friends believes that if she doesn't eat, she'll lose weight. That's not true. You must eat to lose weight. If you don't, your body will think it's starving and burn calories more slowly, which you definitely want to avoid.

If you have a health problem that appears on the following list, you should eliminate coffee and all caffeine in your diet. Caffeine will only exacerbate your condition if you have:

- Acid indigestion, heartburn, or reflux
- Anxiety, irritability, or nervousness
- Candida or yeast problems
- Chronic fatigue syndrome or other autoimmune disorders
- Colitis, diverticulitis, diarrhea, or other irritable bowel symptoms
- Diabetes or hypoglycemia (low blood sugar)
- Dizziness
- Gout
- Heart disease or heart palpitations
- High blood pressure
- High cholesterol
- Insomnia or poor-quality sleep
- Liver disease or gall bladder problems such as gallstones
- Kidney or bladder problems including kidney stones
- Migraines or other vascular headaches
- Osteoporosis
- Skin irritations, rashes, or dryness
- Ulcers or stomach problems such as hiatal hernias
- Urinary tract irritation

To boost your willpower and help you break your addiction, I want to review the health problems associated with consuming too much caffeine. Understanding that caffeine would break down my health over time as it built up in my body made me determined to conquer my dependence. I know heightened awareness will do the same for you. Here is the bad news about caffeine.

Emotional Roller Coaster Ride

Though caffeine can make you anxious and irritable, too much can result in depression and attention disorders. When the caffeine rush wears off, you can crash and feel let down or depressed. To pump yourself up again, you reach for another cup of coffee or can of cola. When you give up caffeine, you might feel a little low for a couple of days. I did, but evening out the peaks and valleys is worth it.

Stress Spike

Caffeine turns on the stress hormones cortisol and adrenaline, which can produce anxiety, irritability, muscular tension and pain, indigestion, insomnia, and decreased immunity. Stress wears you down.

The stress response actually decreases bloodflow to the brain by as much as 30 percent. The reduction of energy available to the brain is not great for memory and mental functioning, which none of us can afford as we get older.

An Alarm That Won't Turn Off

Your adrenal glands produce adrenaline, one of the stress hormones, also known as epinephrine, which sets off the fight-or-flight response. With chronic stress, your adrenals constantly churn out adrenaline. It's as if an alarm is sounding and won't turn off. The emergency stress response elevates your heart rate and increases your respiration and blood pressure so that you can escape danger. Emotional stress elicits the same response even though there is no physical threat. Your adrenal glands reach an exhausted state and stop responding. You become less resistant to stress, and your body stops fighting the invaders, which makes you more vulnerable to hazards like environmental pollutants and disease.

Heart Problems

Caffeine increases your heart rate and elevates your blood pressure, which contributes to the development of heart disease. Regular coffee and decaf increase your cholesterol and homocysteine levels. That means you increase your chance of heart attacks and strokes if your caffeine intake is excessive. Caffeine is also linked to coronary vasospasms, which cause 20 percent of all fatal heart attacks that kill perfectly healthy people. This is important, because heart attacks are often fatal for women who have never been diagnosed with heart disease.

Chock-Full of Acid

More than 208 acids in coffee can contribute to making your body acidic. For optimal health, your body should be alkaline. Much of the Clean Up Your Act

Plan is designed to bring your body back into balance. Over-acidity is associated with health problems that include: weight gain, obesity, loss of skin elasticity (better known as wrinkles), joint pain, loss of vitality, aching muscles, stomachache, ulcers, nausea, urinary tract problems, kidney stones, constipation, gout, osteopenia and osteoporosis, immune deficiency, constriction of blood vessels, and cardiovascular weakness. Are coffee and soda worth it?

Sugar Surges and Crashes

Caffeine stimulates the liver to release glycogen into the bloodstream and creates a sugar surge. The pancreas responds to the rise in blood sugar by releasing insulin, the hormone that causes blood sugar to be stored as fat, something you probably want to avoid. In an hour or two, your blood sugar crashes, and your body is in a state of hypoglycemia or low blood sugar. You feel tired, crave sweets and carbs, grab another cup of coffee, and start the whole cycle over. Caffeinated drinks, even no-cal sodas, trigger the same response. Yes, soda makes you fat.

Ulcers and Reflux

Drinking coffee increases the secretion of hydrochloric acid in your stomach, which can lead to developing ulcers.

Both decaf and coffee reduce the pressure on the valve between the esophagus and the stomach, which allows the highly acidic contents of the stomach to pass up to the esophagus, resulting in heartburn, reflux, and ulcers, and can lead to stomach cancer.

Almost all caffeinated beverages and energy drinks have phosphoric acid added to the sugar water as a preservative. These drinks are extremely acidic and should be avoided.

PMS, Hot Flashes, and Other Female Complaints

Caffeine aggravates a host of female complaints: fibrocystic breast disease, PMS, menopausal problems like hot flashes, osteoporosis, infertility, miscarriage, and low-birth-weight babies. And if you are taking birth control pills, you have a decreased ability to detoxify caffeine.

Reduced Absorption

Caffeine prevents the absorption of some minerals necessary for good health. Those important minerals—including calcium, magnesium, potassium, iron, and trace minerals—are excreted when you urinate. Calcium and magnesium maintain healthy bones and teeth and prevent osteoporosis, especially in post-menopausal women. Reduced calcium absorption is responsible for joint problems and shrinking as you age.

Speeds Up Aging

By the time you are in your thirties, the production of melatonin, DHEA, and other key hormones begins to decline. Melatonin is the pacemaker for your aging clock; DHEA counters the aging effects of menopause. Caffeine hastens the drop. I know I want to keep those hormones as high as possible.

Caffeine slows your cells' ability to repair themselves, which is a fundamental definition of aging. Caffeine also dehydrates the body, which shows on your skin, and inhibits your kidneys from working well. Most important for the purposes of the detox you are about to do, caffeine slows the ability of the liver to detoxify.

You might think I'm laying it on heavy, but I am not exaggerating. Everything you put into your body has an effect. That coffee habit is not doing you any good, except giving you a moment of pleasure. Is it worth it? I don't think so. I

REAL TIME CHANGE

I mostly missed drinking wine, and I can always have a glass of wine every now and then. Frankly, I can have whatever I want—but I want to feel good, so I will remain on the plan.

LUCILLE IRCHA
NEW YORK, NEW YORK

ME: You've got the right idea! The Clean Up Your Act Diet is not about deprivation—it's about making the right choices because you want to feel terrific in the morning.

get a lot of joy watching the birds from my window. I even bought binoculars and an Audubon Guide to see who's in my yard. Appreciating nature will give you more joy and won't cost you your health. Reach for herbal tea when you get the urge to have a hot cup of coffee.

HERE'S TO YOUR HEALTH!

That toast is wishful thinking if you're toasting with alcohol. I've never been much of a drinker, except for my Saturday night lychee martinis, of course. I've seen what alcohol can do to people. It's not pretty. I'm sure you've read that alcohol can reduce the risk of heart disease and maybe do the same for stroke and diabetes. My time in the wine business made me more than familiar with the industry's pitch about the health benefits of drinking. The beneficial effects of alcohol apply to moderate drinking, which is defined for women as one drink a day. One drink a day equals 12 ounces of beer, 5 ounces of wine, or 1.5 ounces of hard liquor. I don't know many people who stop at one drink, do you?

Drinking too much—on a single occasion or over time—can take a serious toll on your body. You probably think of liver disease and injuries from accidents as the main health risks posed by drinking. **The fact is that drinking alcohol has been linked to more than 60 diseases.** Alcohol can affect your body in very destructive ways.

Brain

Alcohol disrupts the brain's communication pathways and can affect the way the brain works. If you have ever watched someone who is extremely drunk, or have been there yourself, you can make a good guess at the areas of the brain that are vulnerable. They include:

- Motor coordination
- Memory
- Emotional response
- The ability to think and plan intelligently
- Social interaction

Heart

Drinking a lot over a long time or bingeing can damage the heart, causing any of the following problems:

- Arrhythmia—irregular heartbeat
- Cardiomyopathy—stretching and drooping of the heart muscle
- Stroke
- High blood pressure

Liver

You are doing the cleanse to help your liver get rid of toxins in your body. After you have been living clean, why would you backpedal? The liver breaks down most of the alcohol you consume and is especially vulnerable to damage from too much drinking. The process generates toxins more harmful than the alcohol itself. These by-products damage liver cells, promote inflammation, and weaken the natural defenses of the body. Heavy drinking can lead to:

- **Fatty liver,** the earliest stage of liver disease. The excessive fat makes it harder for the liver to operate and can lead to inflammation that becomes . . .
- **Alcoholic hepatitis,** which enlarges the liver over time and causes jaundice
- **Fibrosis** causes scar tissue to build up in the liver, which leads to . . .
- **Cirrhosis,** a slow deterioration of the liver

Pancreas

Alcohol causes the pancreas to produce toxic substances that can lead to pancreatitis, a dangerous inflammation and swelling of the blood vessels in the pancreas that prevents proper digestion.

Cancer

Drinking too much alcohol has been found to increase your risk of developing certain cancers, including:

- Mouth
- Esophagus
- Throat
- Liver
- Breast

Immune System

Drinking too much can weaken your immune system, making your body susceptible to disease. Habitual drinkers are more likely to develop pneumonia and tuberculosis than people who drink only occasionally. A night of binge drinking can compromise your body's ability to fight off infections—even up to 24 hours after getting drunk. This is why you are not supposed to drink alcohol if you have a bacterial or viral infection.

And There Are More Reasons Not to Drink

Social drinking leads to nibbling unhealthy, salty things and sabotages your willpower. People eat more when they drink.

Alcohol also disrupts your sleep. It's hard enough to get a full night's sleep once you approach menopause.

The dehydrating effect of alcohol will show on your face. Aging will take its toll naturally. You don't need to give it a hand by drinking.

Giving up alcohol is not easy if you are accustomed to having a glass of wine or a cocktail to unwind after a hectic day, to celebrate, to accompany a good meal, or to kill the pain of a boring social event. I have a friend who drives me crazy. She refuses to do the cleanse, because she won't give up alcohol. She doesn't think she can get through a day without a drink. Her martinis mean more to her than her health. She's totally unwilling to take control of her own

> **REAL TIME CHANGE**
>
> I reminded myself that if we are able to refrain from having alcohol for 9 months while pregnant plus whatever months we are breastfeeding, we should most certainly be able to do this. If we're able to adopt healthier choices for the sake of our unborn babies, we should find the strength to do it for ourselves as well.
>
> ILIANA GUIBERT
NEW YORK, NEW YORK
>
> ME: Brilliant! Now you're talking. There's nothing like a mother's strength.

life. A martini is the boss of her. She can't face 2 weeks without booze. I'm on her case all the time just to try the cleanse to see how much better she would feel emotionally and physically when she says no to a habit that will only hurt her in the long run.

If you think about your health over the long term, the perspective of what you can prevent should make cutting back or completely eliminating your consumption of alcohol something you want to do. You have the power to do anything you want. Don't forget it!

Now you know the reasons for staying away from processed food, sugar, GMOs, traditionally raised produce and livestock, gluten, dairy, caffeine, and alcohol to clean up your act. What you've learned in this chapter should confirm that you made the right decision by committing to change the way you eat. Your goals are clear. You are no longer lost in the maze. You have a path to follow, like the yellow brick road. As long as you know the way, you just have to put one foot in front of the other. You can do this!

In the end, only three things matter: how much you loved, how gently you lived, and how gracefully you let go of things not meant for you.
—FROM *BUDDHA'S LITTLE INSTRUCTION BOOK* BY JACK KORNFIELD

An overburdened liver sounds different from a healthy one. An overburdened liver groans. It groans and begs. It begs for a day off. A day to deal with the worst of the garbage. The way things are now, it's always in a hurry, trying to catch up with itself. The overburdened liver is like the kitchen in a restaurant that's open around the clock. The dishes pile up. The dishwashers are working full tilt. But the dirty dishes and caked-on pans only pile up higher and higher. The overburdened liver hopes for that one day off that never comes.
—FROM THE NOVEL *SUMMER HOUSE WITH SWIMMING POOL* BY HERMAN KOCH

CHAPTER

5

Cleaning from the Inside Out

You have decided to do a good thing by giving your liver the break it needs to catch up with the backlog of garbage that has accumulated. The best way to begin cleaning up your act is to start from the inside out by detoxifying your body. The 14-Day Liver Cleanse that transformed me will put you on a fast track to optimal health. **When you activate all the detox pathways in your body and** flush out the toxins that have been building up your entire life, you are ready to make a fresh start and jump-start change. You will feel the positive effects in just 3 or 4 days. By the end of the 2-week cleanse, you will be purified and feeling so good that you'll want to stay that way. You are going to be surprised at how easy this is. The thought of doing a cleanse seemed so challenging to me, but actually doing it was a snap. Take my word for it—you are going to breeze through this. I'll walk you through the program step-by-step. In the Real Time Change sidebars, words from women who have completed the program and made huge changes in their diets will support and motivate you. We're giving you the tools to take control of your well-being.

REAL TIME CHANGE

I feel clean, from the inside out. Most interesting and important, I feel calm—calm about my body, about its ability to direct to a normal, natural weight, and what it needs to achieve a healthy state. My old definitions of what a healthy state was have finally been changed. I feel certain my body is happy about that!

What a recalibration! I was in it for the weight loss, but the outcome was much different than I expected. I learned to trust that my body knows its healthy weight. Eating clean gave me that lesson.

This is the easiest, most manageable program a professional dieter like myself can maintain.

DIANE ARPINO
RAMSEY, NEW JERSEY

ME: You've learned such an important lesson about your body's ability to take care of itself if you feed it well. Now you don't have to mess up your body's balance with every diet that comes along. You have a plan that works.

If you have any of the nagging physical problems that are listed below, cleansing your liver will probably help:

- Overweight/underweight
- Fatigue
- Insomnia

- Frequent flus, colds, sinus infections
- Muscle and joint pain
- Dark circles under your eyes
- Constipation
- Bloating
- Diarrhea
- Nausea
- Heartburn
- Allergies
- Chemical sensitivities
- Elevated cholesterol
- PMS

Even if you don't have symptoms yet, a lifetime's accumulation of damaging toxins from the environment, the food you eat, the furnishings in your house or apartment, and the personal grooming products you use takes its toll on your health. You know about the toxins in the air you breathe. You don't have much control over the polluted air outside. But did you know that there are much higher concentrations of 20 toxic compounds in your home than there are outdoors? You heard me: The air in your house or apartment can be more toxic than the air in polluted cities. The materials used in modern construction, the furnishings, and the chemicals in cleaning products all contribute to your toxic load. There are 15,000 chemical ingredients used in personal grooming products, and 90 percent of those chemicals have never been tested. The average woman uses 515 chemical ingredients a day on her body. Every time you wash your hair, put on hand cream, "protect" your lips with gloss, and have a mani-pedi, you are exposing yourself to powerful toxins.

DETOXING IS NOT OPTIONAL—IT'S NECESSARY

Toxins, toxins everywhere! There's no escaping. We are virtually bombarded with harmful chemicals in every aspect of our lives. More than 80,000 man-made chemicals have been introduced since World War II. Your body does not experience these toxins one at a time. No one knows the effects of the

Toxic Surprises

Aside from the toxins in your food and the pollution in the environment, you are exposed to toxins every day that you may not be aware of. When you consider pollution, you probably think about the earth's atmosphere, soil, and water. You understand that industrial waste and car emissions do a lot of damage, but live unaware of the toxic stew in your own home. The clothes you wear, the mattress you sleep on, the finish on your floors, your lipstick, and the shampoo, soap, and toothpaste you use contain highly toxic ingredients. Here are just a few examples of toxins to which you are exposed that may not register on your radar.

- The appliances of modern life—cell phones, computers, televisions, and microwaves—disrupt electromagnetic fields and outgas, which means they release or give off toxic gas or vapors containing harmful chemicals.
- House paint contains highly toxic solvents and volatile organic compounds.
- Dry cleaning fluid residues are powerful neurotoxins.
- Synthetic fabrics are petroleum based and processed with many chemicals that can be absorbed through your skin.
- Vinyl flooring is toxic, and polyurethane finishes outgas toxins.
- Plastic food containers, food packaging, and wraps contain highly toxic phthalates and BPA, which are especially toxic when microwaved.

chemical interactions you are exposed to day and night.

You can't live in a bubble. No matter how hard you try, you cannot avoid toxic exposure. You can be a fanatic about what you eat, your grooming products, makeup, and clothes, and try making your home a toxic-free zone, but you will always be exposed to harmful chemicals and substances despite your best efforts to avoid them. **Toxins are inescapable in modern life. Detoxifying your body by cleaning it deeply from the inside out is essential if you want to stay healthy.**

HOW TOXINS MAKE YOU SICK

Though your body is designed to neutralize and eliminate toxins, today there are so many man-made chemicals that the body's ability to process and neutralize

- Carpets and upholstered furniture outgas formaldehyde and other toxins.

- If a product under your sink has a warning label that says "Caution," "May cause skin irritation," "Danger," "Keep out of reach of children," or "Corrosive," you should throw it out. Ninety percent of health problems with highly toxic substances found in household cleaning products are caused by inhalation of vapors and absorption of particles.

- Mattresses contain flame-retardants by law. Those chemicals are neurotoxins.

- Nonstick pots and pans can be deadly, especially if the coating is scratched.

- The fluoride in toothpaste that prevents cavities is a neurotoxin.

- Traces of lead, arsenic, cadmium, and other heavy metals have been found in lipsticks and glosses. These heavy metals are extremely toxic to the nervous system. Synthetic oils, dyes, and petroleum waxes complete the list of toxic ingredients in lipstick and gloss.

- Any clothes that are labeled "permanent press," "no-iron," "wrinkle-resistant," or "stain proof" have been treated with potentially dangerous, untested chemicals that make them easy care.

- Women who have their hair dyed five or more times a year have twice the risk of developing ovarian cancer. Darker dyes pose a greater health risk. Twenty-two ingredients in hair dyes have been banned in Europe, but the toxins have not been restricted in the United States.

  We pay a high price for living in the chemical age.

them can be overwhelmed. When those toxins build up inside your body, they damage your cells, disrupt how your body functions, and compromise your well-being. The term "toxic load" refers to all the contaminants you've been exposed to in your life. Your emotions and stress also affect the mix.

Think of a stockpot on the burner of your stove. It boils over if you add too many ingredients and cook it with too much heat. Your body is like that pot of soup. It will boil over if you add too many toxic substances and heat the pot up with extreme stress. Your body can't handle the toxic burden, and the excessive toxins will make you sick. You might experience vague symptoms like dull hair, headaches, or allergies, as well as the list of nagging physical problems—which are toxic overload symptoms—at the beginning of this chapter. These are symptoms that can indicate your body is slowly being poisoned. If you have these chronic problems and do not lower your body burden, you will get sick. **With toxic overload, your body becomes inflamed and acidic. Your immune system goes into overdrive, reacting nonstop to the presence of toxins by trying to expel them. In an effort to dilute the toxins circulating in your bloodstream, your body retains fluids, and you get bloated. Your body can no longer get rid of the toxins efficiently. Those nagging symptoms eventually develop into full-fledged disease.**

OBESOGENS: SOME TOXINS MAKE IT TOUGH TO LOSE WEIGHT

Scientific research has discovered a class of toxins known as obesogens. They are endocrine disruptors that affect the way the body stores fat and burns energy. These toxins disturb the systems that control your weight. Obesogens increase the number of fat cells you have, decrease the calories you burn, and change the way your body manages hunger. No thank you very much. I am talking about seriously disrupting your metabolism. Even low exposure to the obesogens that follow can promote weight gain.

Pesticides and herbicides found in conventionally farmed crops leach into the soil and run off into the water supply. When you consume meat, poultry, and farm-raised fish that have been fed treated grains, the pesticides are stored in your fat cells. Organic is the way to go.

Hormones and antibiotics, used to fatten livestock and keep them infection-free, accumulate in the animals' fat cells and are passed on to you when you eat conventionally raised beef and poultry. The role of the hormones is to slow down the animals' metabolism so that they gain weight. When you eat meat or poultry treated with these chemicals, your body responds in the same way. The chemicals fatten you up, and the antibiotics can make other antibiotics less effective when you need them.

High-fructose corn syrup is an ingredient in most processed foods. Consuming corn syrup creates a weight-gain cycle: You crave more food that is quickly stored as fat. Eating close to the source will protect you!

BPA (bisphenol A) is used to make plastic hard. It is used in plastic bottles, can linings, thermal paper used for cash register receipts, and electronic devices. The chemical has been found in 93 percent of pregnant American women tested and the babies they carry. BPA increases insulin resistance and has been linked to obesity. Fortunately, manufacturers are starting to produce plastics without BPA—look for the label.

PFOA (perfluorooctanoic acid) is a component of nonstick coatings of pots and pans, of the lining of microwave popcorn bags, and of the finish on stain-resistant fabrics. This compound affects the thyroid hormones. Replace any scratched or worn nonstick pots.

Phthalates are hard-to-avoid plasticizers, commonly found in cosmetics, air fresheners, shower curtains, perfume, food containers, and food packaging. You know that awful smell you sometimes get when you open up something packaged in plastic. I've always thought that if it smells that bad, it can't be good for you! Phthalates have been associated with loss of muscle mass and weight gain.

I'm mentioning only a few of the known obesogens. I'm sure scientists will find hundreds if not thousands more chemicals that are contributing to the obesity epidemic.

Obesogens make losing weight difficult. Toxins stored in fat cells can remain stuck there, because your body is protecting you by resisting the release of these poisons. When you lose weight, fat cells release the stored toxins along with the glucose. The liberated obesogens lower your thyroid hormone levels, which slows down your metabolic rate and reduces further fat burning to keep your body from releasing more toxins back into circulation. The more fat you start with, the more toxins are released. Since your body wants to protect you by storing those toxins as fat, losing additional weight becomes difficult. In other words, losing weight can prevent further weight loss.

The way to stop this frustrating cycle is to detox. Only then will you break through weight plateaus as your body is able to flush out the toxins released with weight loss. That is why I always say that losing weight is a by-product of doing a deep cleanse.

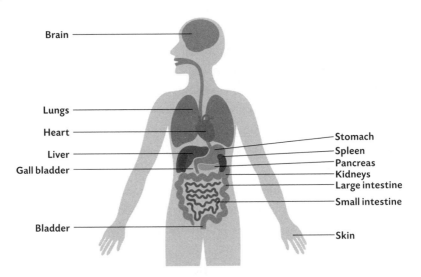

NATURAL DETOX

Your health depends on your body's ability to eliminate toxins from your cells, organs, and bloodstream. Healthy cells automatically detoxify themselves. The process is so important that many interlocking systems operate to do the job. **Your body is a detox machine that processes and expels chemicals and waste materials through your skin, lungs, kidneys, lymphatic system, colon, and liver.** There is a lot going on in that body of yours—you have to change the oil to keep all systems running smoothly. The organs that follow are the working parts of the detox engine.

A Two-Way Street: Skin

Your skin is the largest organ of elimination. Toxins leave your body through perspiration. Sauna, steam, and detox baths promote the excretion of heavy metals like lead and mercury and harmful fat-soluble chemicals. The skin is also an organ of absorption. Putting something on your skin is like eating it. Toxins enter your body through your skin and travel through the bloodstream, damaging cells before the chemicals reach your liver to be filtered out. **When you walk through a drug store or the first floor of a department store, you have a choice of thousands of beauty products. My advice: Pay more attention to the ingredients than to the promises.**

Deep-Breathing Assist: Lungs

Your lungs filter the air, and your breath expels many contaminants when you exhale. The blood carries used and toxic gases to your lungs to be eliminated with each exhalation. Breathing properly is an important part of detoxifying your body. You have to breathe deeply to oxygenate your body and brain. Proper breathing helps keep lymphatic circulation moving to remove cellular waste. To eliminate toxins, you have to keep that lymph fluid moving. Stand up and sit straight and breathe deeply to help your body detox.

The Second Transport System: Lymphatic System

Your body has two circulatory systems: the bloodstream and the lymphatic system. The latter supports the immune system by removing and destroying waste, debris, dead blood cells, pathogens, toxins, and cancer cells. Lymphatic fluid absorbs fat-soluble vitamins from the digestive system and delivers the nutrients to the body's cells. Since the lymphatic system does not have a heart to pump it, its movement depends on the motions of the muscles and joints, which is another reason you have to keep moving. As the lymph fluid moves upward toward the neck, it passes through the lymph nodes, which filter it to remove waste and pathogens. Lymphatic massage can help remove toxins from your body. Brushing your body when you bathe is also helpful.

Flush Out Toxins: Kidneys

The kidneys filter and recirculate blood to flush out waste. They need plenty of water to do the job. A well-hydrated body produces urine that is mostly clear with only a slight tinge of yellow. If your urine has a strong odor or is dark in color, you are not drinking enough water. **Water is a vehicle for detoxing. The water you drink should not contribute to your toxic load. Stick to bottled or filtered water.**

Clean and Clear: Colon

The colon receives solid waste from the rest of the body. When the colon is not doing its job, waste backs up into the bloodstream. To make up for the colon's inability to expel toxins, the other organs of elimination have to work harder. When dead material backs up in the colon, bacteria, viruses, molds, and parasites feed on the waste matter, which they break down. The immune system kicks in to help with elimination, and your body becomes inflamed to kill off and remove the germs. When your immune system is overwhelmed, disease sets in. Keeping your colon clean and clear is a crucial element of good health. This is why fiber is so important. Get ready to eat a lot of vegetables and fruit!

Detox Central: Liver

Your health and well-being are closely linked to the health of your liver. A major processing plant with more than 600 functions, the liver is a vital organ that responds to the demands of the body by shifting blood to specific areas. The liver stores blood sugar as glycogen and releases it into the bloodstream when needed. The liver regulates insulin production, controls fat metabolism, and makes cholesterol. **The liver is also a detox plant. It filters poisons in the bloodstream, neutralizes them, and sends them on to the other elimination organs.**

When the liver becomes overloaded, toxins pass through the filter a few times, damaging cells until the liver can neutralize the harmful chemicals. This extra strain reduces the liver's ability to do other jobs, resulting in high cholesterol, imbalanced hormones, unregulated blood sugar, and raised blood pressure. An overloaded liver leads to inflammation. When excess toxins overwhelm the liver, they can be redeposited in the joints or as plaque on the walls of blood vessels and the intestines, held in cysts, or lodged in fatty areas of the brain, breast, or prostate.

REAL TIME CHANGE

I feel like a new person. This was the best thing I have done for myself in a long time. I took my blood pressure, and even though I'm on medication, it is usually high. My pressure was 128/83, which is really good for me. I am a person who used to get stomachaches a lot. I have not had one stomachache since doing the cleanse.

DALE LAWRENCE
DANVERS, MASSACHUSETTS

ME: And you thought you were doing this to lose weight! This cleanse is so much more than that. We don't have to assume that high blood pressure and digestive problems are an inevitable part of aging. You don't have to sit back and accept uncomfortable physical symptoms. Don't view aches and pains as a part of aging. You have the power to change all that.

Think of your liver as a mop that cleans up toxins. You have to squeeze that mop out now and then if you want it to do its job and not become a soggy mess. Your liver is the crucial target of the cleanse you will be doing. A healthy liver will keep you clean inside. Once your liver is clean, losing weight will be easier. Instead of being slogged down, your liver will be able to work overtime to filter the toxins released from your fat cells as your body burns the energy stored in your fat and gets rid of them.

WHAT HAPPENS WHEN YOU DO A LIVER CLEANSE

Detoxing the liver happens in two phases. This chemical process is not to be confused with the three stages of your liver cleanse, which are based on what you do on the program. **The first phase process breaks down toxins; the second phase makes them easy to flush out.** Most of the toxins to which you are exposed are fat soluble. They are absorbed by the fatty part of cells instead of being excreted in water-based urine. When toxins settle into cells, they exert their toxic effects on the liver, colon, kidneys, heart, brain, lungs, skin, and hormones. A good cleanse assists the liver in changing harmful fat-soluble toxins into a water-soluble form that can be eliminated from the body. The liver goes through a two-step process to break down toxins into harmless substances.

PHASE 1 OF A LIVER DETOXIFICATION
(Days 1 to 7 of the Cleanse)

This is the liver's first defense against toxic chemical compounds. A group of enzymes attack fat-soluble toxins and change them. The substances that are formed from these reactions are more toxic than the original toxins, which is why you might not feel well at the beginning of the cleanse. If the products of this action are not further reduced into less harmful substances, these toxins can accumulate and cause allergies, frequent colds and flus, and other illnesses. But you don't have to worry about that. There's a Phase 2 to get rid of those toxins.

Nutrients Needed for Phase 1

These nutrients, which are present in abundance in the supplements you will be taking, help your liver to break down toxins.

Vitamins B_2, B_3, B_6, B_{12}	Folic acid
Glutathione	Flavonoids

PHASE 2 OF A LIVER DETOXIFICATION
(Days 8 to 14 of the Cleanse)

Now your body will shift into a deeper cleanse by processing the altered toxins for elimination. In this stage, the liver converts the products of Phase 1 into nontoxic molecules that are excreted from your body through urine, bile, or stool. This process is accomplished by attaching molecules to the highly toxic compounds to neutralize them. Six detoxification pathways convert the products of Phase 1 so that your body can easily eliminate the toxic waste. If the information that follows is more than you want to know, skip it. I find that if I can visualize what is going on inside my body, I am even more motivated to follow the plan, so here goes.

1. **Sulfation:** This is the main liver detox pathway that attaches sulfur-containing compounds to the products of Phase 1. This pathway neutralizes the stress hormone cortisol as well as some prescription medicines, food additives, environmental toxins, and intestinal bacteria that produce toxins.

2. **Glucuronidation:** Glucuronic acid combines with toxins to detoxify certain medications—aspirin, for example—food additives and preservatives, and reproductive and adrenal hormones. Magnesium also supports this process.

3. **Glutathione:** The attachment of glutathione to toxins helps to eliminate fat-soluble toxins, especially heavy metals like mercury and lead. Glutathione is a very important antioxidant and anticancer agent. Nutrients that help to increase levels of glutathione include vitamin C, alpha-lipoic acid, and the amino acids glutamine and methionine.

4. **Acetylation:** Acetyl CoA attaches to toxins to make them less harmful and easy to excrete. For this pathway to work at its optimal level, vitamins B_5 and C are needed.

5. **Amino acid conjugation:** Glycine, taurine, and glutamine attach to toxins in this pathway. These amino acids help the body to excrete many toxic chemicals from the body. Amino acids are found in protein-rich foods.

6. **Methylation:** Methyl groups attach to toxins, particularly steroid hormones like estrogen. Methionine drives this pathway, which needs vitamin B_{12}, folic acid, and choline to function properly.

Nutrients Needed for Phase 2

The following list of nutrients will give your body a big assist in neutralizing and flushing out the toxins from your body.

Methionine	Cysteine
Glycine	Magnesium
Taurine	Glutathione
Glutamine	Vitamin B_5, B_{12}
Folic acid	Vitamin C
Choline	

TIME FOR SPRING CLEANING

Fortunately, you can relieve the stress on your liver, rev up the elimination of toxins, and stimulate the release of obesogens by doing the 14-Day Liver Cleanse I describe in the next chapter. Your goal is to drastically reduce and wipe clean a lifetime of exposure. When you think of the cleanse that way, committing just 2 weeks seems like nothing. You can rally to do just about anything for 14 days. Reducing your toxic burden will put you on the path to optimal health. Lowering your toxic load will give your body a break and allow it to direct energy to healing. By following the program, you will be living and eating in a way that will dramatically reduce your exposure to the toxins you can control. This cleanse will reenergize your exhausted, overwhelmed liver and restore it to being a super toxin elimination plant. You can't imagine how much a sluggish liver affects the way you look and feel. Every other system in your body is compromised if your liver is not functioning properly. By boosting your body's natural ability to detoxify, you will begin to experience remarkable changes in only 2 weeks.

One of the side benefits of this cleanse, besides weight loss, is improved digestion. Removing harmful toxins from your body will boost nutrient absorption, and that's the secret to having super energy. For maximum effect, you have to carry on after the cleanse with my Clean Up Your Act Diet, but that is something you'll be happy to do when you see how great you feel after you clean your

REAL TIME CHANGE

For me, this was a new lease on life and another chance at feeling wonderful. The word I have used to describe how I feel to my friends is "euphoric."

I have tried other products, diets, and fads in the past, all resulting in failure. I can honestly say that this has been great and easy for me. I never thought I would have the willpower. I wish I could get everyone on this to see what a change in your life it would make.

JEANIE CIUPPA SANTACROCE
LODI, NEW JERSEY

ME: Well, that's what I'm trying to do. When you find something that works, you want everyone to know about it.

house from top to bottom. When you've finished your spring cleaning, everything is in order, as fresh and new as the weather outside. You can choose to do the same for your body. You can refresh yourself from the inside out and be invigorated by a sense of purpose and accomplishment.

The cleanse is not just physical. As you cleanse your body of toxins, you should clear your mind of negative patterns and set a new course. Make sure gratitude and appreciation of life are on your daily menu. Choose to savor life—a meal, a smile, a conversation, a moment. Be aware of the beauty that exists everywhere. Take it all in! Your life will be richer if you do.

You are ready for action! The first moves you make will be nitty-gritty preparations for the cleanse. It's time to get organized so that your cleanse will be hassle free.

CHAPTER

6

Cleanse Prep

I bet by now you're wondering, "Is she ever going to tell me what I have to do?" The buildup is all part of the plan! I'm glad you're chomping at the bit like a thoroughbred racehorse. I want you fired up to take control, now that you've learned to think about food another way. I've set you up for success by convincing you that this 14-day cleanse is about a lot more than losing weight. It's a race every one of you can win. I'm thrilled for you as you take your place at the starting gate. You have an exciting ride ahead.

THE 14-DAY LIVER CLEANSE

This is the simple cleanse that saved my life. It has three stages:

Stage 1: Fasting (Days 1 and 2). You will have a protein shake in the morning and evening and will take two multivitamin/mineral capsules without iron in the morning and again in the evening. You read it right—no solid food for 2 days. To my surprise, I wasn't hungry at all.

83

Stage 2: Reintroducing Solid Food (Days 3 to 7). You will continue to have two protein shakes and two multivitamins/minerals, and will add two phytonutrient capsules in the morning and again at night. Meal plans and recipes will ease you back into eating solid food so that your digestive system is not strained.

Stage 3: Boosting Toxin Elimination (Days 8 to 14). You will add another phytonutrient in the morning and evening to the supplements you are taking. So you will have a protein shake, two multivitamins/minerals, and three phytonutrients in the morning and again in the evening. We have included meal plans and recipes for Stage 3.

The Clean Up Your Act Diet. After your 14-Day Liver Cleanse, you will begin the Clean Up Your Act Diet with guidelines for how to eat for the rest of your life. Two weeks of meal plans are included to launch you into a new way of eating.

THE SUPPLEMENTS

The week before you begin the cleanse, you should purchase your supplements. Build in enough time to allow for shipping if necessary. We recommend that you start the cleanse on a Friday for reasons I will explain later.

I think it is important for you to be confident that the three supplements you will be taking will be effective nutritional supports for your cleanse and will provide you with everything you need to detoxify successfully. I wanted to be certain that the products we recommended were as natural and effective as they could be, so I developed Liv4Mor, my own line of supplements with Lisa. I know they are very effective. Of course, there are many fine products out there that will gently support your body's unique cleansing process. We will suggest the best products available to help you cleanse successfully.

You should purchase a 2-week supply of protein shake powder, multivitamins/minerals without iron (56 capsules), and phytonutrients (62 capsules).

Shake Powders

Protein shake powder can be mixed with water, rice milk, or almond milk, but I definitely recommend using rice or almond milk. A shake made with water tastes yucky. Speaking of yucky reminds me to warn you to drink the shake as soon as you make it. Some shakes get glutinous as the fiber swells. If you leave it even for a short time, you will be grossed out. The blend of protein, fiber, and nutrients in the protein shake powder will help eliminate toxins. Vegetable proteins are the way to go. Since you will not be eating dairy, whey protein is not for you. Your drink should also provide the fiber needed to bind toxins for elimination.

Lisa is an advocate of protein powders that are created from the ground up. By that she means a protein powder based in plants—seeds, fruits, and vegetables. Typically, pea, brown rice, and hemp proteins are combined to produce a mixed plant-based protein formula that provides a variety of nutrients in one powder. The powder should contain minerals, greens, and antioxidants. We recommend the following protein shakes:

Liv4Mor Cleanse Powder uses organic, whole-grain brown rice protein that will fill you up and give you an allergy-free source of energy. Other ingredients include N-acetyl cysteine along with glycine and taurine, amino acids known to support the liver. The unique blend of vegetable extracts includes broccoli sprout concentrate, onion extract, tomato, broccoli, carrot, spinach, kale, and Brussels sprouts, providing natural antioxidants. Powerful antioxidants like lipoic acid, green tea, and ellagic acid work synergistically with the vegetable antioxidant blend to help the liver in the detoxification process.

Vega One All-in-One Nutritional Shake: Combines pea, brown rice, hemp seed, and sacha inchi proteins. This plant-based powder also includes the superfoods flaxseeds and chia seeds for omega-3s.

22 Days Plant Protein Power: The blend in this powder is made up of organic fruits and vegetables and flaxseeds.

Sunwarrior Blend Raw Vegan Protein: raw, gluten-free vegan protein

Garden of Life Raw Meal Beyond Organic Meal Replacement: raw, vegan, gluten free, and dairy free

Multivitamin/Mineral Capsules without Iron

The multivitamin/mineral capsules without iron should be comprehensive multivitamins that provide key minerals and nutrients that support detoxification. High levels of antioxidants reduce free radical damage. Look for multivitamins without iron. The reason for not taking iron is that the body has no way to eliminate excess iron, which accumulates in the tissues and organs, especially the liver. Too much iron can cause liver scarring, which can lead to cirrhosis in some cases. Since you are trying to detox your liver, you do not want to add to its work.

You will need 56 capsules for the 2-week cleanse. My recommended multivitamin/mineral capsules are:

Liv4Mor Multivitamins and Minerals without Iron

Nature's Way Alive! Whole Food Energizer Multi-Vitamin Max Potency No Added Iron

Whole Foods 365 Adult Multi Vitamin

Solaray Once Daily High Energy Multi-Vita-Min

New Chapter Only One Whole-Food Multivitamin

Rainbow Light Active Adult 50+ Multivitamin

Rainbow Light Just Once Iron-Free Multivitamin (VeganGuard, gluten free)

Phytonutrients

Phytonutrients, which are found in plants, help eliminate toxins and stimulate the liver during your detox. They are believed to protect your health by serving as antioxidants, enhancing your body's ability to fight off disease, improving cell-to-cell communication, repairing damage to DNA caused by exposure to toxins, and detoxifying carcinogens that lead to cancer.

You will need 62 capsules for the two-week cleanse. These are the best on the market for the purpose of your cleanse.

Liv4Mor Phytonutrients. Its natural botanicals boost the liver's cleansing function. For example, silymarin (milk thistle extract) is used to protect the liver from medications and environmental contaminants. Silymarin, along with curcumin and radish root, increase enzyme activity in the liver. Artichoke, yellow dock, and dandelion root stimulate production of bile in the liver.

Nature's Way Super Thisilyn Liver Support Advanced Detox Formula

Renew Life Liver Detox 30-Day Program

Whole Foods 365 Complete Body Cleanse, 2 week or 30 Day Plan

GET RID OF THE JUNK IN YOUR KITCHEN CABINETS

Take the time to sort through the food in your pantry. Get rid of cookies, cake mixes, bread, rolls, muffins, crackers, candy, salty snacks, processed food of every type, pasta, sauces in jars, jellies and jams with sugar, relishes, sodas, ketchup, sugar, sugar substitutes, flour, coffee, caffeinated tea, converted and white rice, flavored rice mixes, taco shells, salad dressings, barbecue sauces, pancake mix, and all oils but extra virgin olive oil and raw coconut oil. Do the same in your freezer and refrigerator. Get rid of frozen prepared meals, ice cream, frozen yogurt, low-calorie pops, butter, margarine, milk, cream, and yogurt. These foods are no longer part of your diet. There are a lot of hungry people in the world who would benefit from having any food at all. Make a donation of the food you won't be eating to food drives or charitable organizations. A list of the foods that are and are not on the plan appears on pages 106 and 107.

Organize your dried herbs and spices, because you will be relying on them in your new approach to food. You will be eating natural food that is not loaded with salt, sugar, and fat. The flavors you will be enjoying are more subtle than the overkill taste of processed foods. Herbs and spices will become key ingredients in the food you eat.

I was able to skip this process when I did my first cleanse, because I had just moved into a new house and the cupboards were bare. I started from scratch, which was ideal. I'm happy to report that I have very little in my kitchen cabinets 4 years later. When your diet consists of simple, fresh food, you don't need to keep a lot on hand. It's liberating to see all that space.

If you have a family to feed, who are not ready to change their eating habits, clear a shelf for yourself so that you can isolate your food. When you buy food for your family, you should avoid things that you love. Don't add more temptation. There is always another cookie or ice-cream flavor. As your family eats their way through the not-so-healthy food in your pantry, you can gradually replace the junk with healthy food. Your family might become converts as they watch you change day by day and see the delicious food you are preparing for yourself. After all, there's nothing like a home-cooked meal. Now that you've left prepared food behind, that's how you'll be eating. It won't be long before your family sees the value—and pleasure—of eating clean.

REAL TIME CHANGE

Once I transformed my cabinets and refrigerator to accommodate the everyday clean eating plan, it was easy. My family has been extremely supportive and, for the most part, they have started eating clean themselves! We are all trying new things and recipes. I recently purchased a CSA (community supported agriculture) share at a local farm, and every Wednesday I pick up my "share" of organic seasonal vegetables and fruits.

LORETTA LANG STOKES
BEVERLY, MASSACHUSETTS

ME: Supporting local farmers is a good thing! What you are eating is as fresh as it can be. How great it is that you have the support of your family.

Eating new things is good. I never even knew what quinoa was, and now it's one of my favorite foods.

YOUR NEW FOOD PANTRY

The week before your cleanse, you should stock your kitchen cabinets with the staples of your new diet. Since so much of what you eat will be fresh, you will not need a lot of space. Here are some of the nonperishable food items you should have on hand.

- Almond butter
- Almond milk
- Bottled water and/or a water filter jug or system
- Brown rice
- Cans of organic beans—chickpeas (garbanzo beans), black beans, kidney beans, great Northern beans
- Cans of organic tomatoes
- Capers
- Celtic sea salt
- Chia seeds
- Dried beans if you prefer them to canned
- Extra virgin olive oil

- Gluten-free crackers
- Herbal teas
- Lentils—red and green (they cook up quickly)
- Low-sodium organic stocks—beef, chicken, and vegetable
- Mustards
- Quinoa—in a variety of colors
- Raw almonds, walnuts, cashews, pumpkin seeds
- Raw coconut oil
- Rice cakes
- Rice milk
- Tahini
- Vinegars

For the detox baths in your future:

- Epsom salts
- Big bag of baking soda
- Aromatherapy oil
- A bath brush

While you are fasting, you will buy the fresh produce and meat you will be eating for the balance of the cleanse. That list appears in the next chapter.

KEEP A FOOD JOURNAL

During your 2-week trial, I recommend keeping a daily journal to record what you are eating, how much exercise you are getting, and how you are feeling. Write it all down on your phone, on the computer, or in a special notebook. Doing so will help you to stay on track. You will gain an understanding of your typical rhythms during the day and see how you are progressing. Write about when you feel challenged. Is it hard to follow the cleanse in social situations? Are you able to handle it eating out?

Aside from keeping track of your cleanse, you might go through changes in your emotions and attitudes. You should capture how you are feeling as you progress through the cleanse. Is your mood lighter? Are you calmer? Keeping a record will encourage you to make healthy choices in your life. Paying attention to your emotions, self-esteem, and capacity to stop and smell the roses will give

DAILY LOG

How did you feel upon waking up?

How many hours did you sleep? And how well?

Breakfast:

When did you get hungry, and how hungry were you on a scale of 1 to 10, with 10 being ravenous?

Midmorning snack:

When did you get hungry and how hungry (1–10)?

Lunch:

When did you get hungry and how hungry (1–10)?

Midafternoon snack:

When did you get hungry and how hungry (1–10)?

How did you feel before dinner?

Dinner:

How hungry were you before bed (1–10):

you an idea of the emotional healing going on as you eliminate poisons from your body. Here are some questions to consider when you are recording your experience of the cleanse.

How did you feel before bed?

Cups of fluid: ❏ ❏ ❏ ❏ ❏ ❏ ❏ ❏

How long did you exercise, what did you do, and when did you do it?

When was your energy highest today?

When was your energy lowest today?

Did you have any cravings during the day? If so, how did you deal with it?

What do you miss eating or drinking the most?

Have you noticed any effect on your emotions?

Have you seen a change in your physical complaints?

Did you have a hard time eating this way with friends and family?

Did friends and family support you?

When did you start to notice a difference in how you felt and looked?

Have others noticed a change in you? When?

REAL TIME CHANGE

New skill set for me: food journaling. I always tried to get in the habit before! For some reason, I never kept up with food journaling. This time, I didn't go crazy writing, but I did track my behavior, etc. I don't know if it was the inspirational kickoff, the camaraderie, or the solid goals we set, but the liver cleanse felt like a fresh starting point to journaling. I saw results, which really helped me to journal. There was a whole new dimension of improving my future quality of life that was motivating. So I was not just recording what I ate and how I felt, I was analyzing it. It really blew me away to realize that many times I wanted to eat out of habit not hunger.

HELYN L. BRYANT
HILLCREST, NEW YORK

ME: Keeping a journal is a big support as you start on a program that will change your life. It's great to capture the moment, to have a day-by-day record of your transformation. When you do the cleanse again, you will be able to compare the experiences. I think the cleanse goes deeper each time you do it.

JUMP-START CHANGE

When Lisa puts people on the cleanse, she asks them to have before-and-after blood tests done. Comparing the blood work gives them hard proof of their improved health. It's remarkable to see the changes that happen in just 2 weeks. You might want to do the same. When you see the direct effect of what you are doing, you'll be convinced that you can take charge of your health.

Lisa has learned, after putting hundreds of people on this cleanse, that it is a good idea to begin the program at the end of the week, because you may be slightly uncomfortable for a couple of days. I had a headache during the fasting days and was very tired. You may have flulike symptoms, body aches, nausea, and mood changes. **During the 2-day fast, the symptoms and their intensity vary from person to person depending on how much toxic burden you are carrying. The good news is that if you are feeling off, there is a great reason for it. Your body is cleaning house, releasing stored toxins into your blood-**

stream to be flushed away. Won't you be glad to get rid of those poisons? These symptoms are only temporary. If you are concerned about how your body is reacting, contact your health care provider. Starting Stage 1, your 2-day fast, on a Friday will make any discomfort you may be feeling easier to handle. Days 2 and 3 tend to be when people doing the cleanse feel the worst, so plan to spend a quiet weekend.

The first time I did the cleanse in January 4 years ago, Lisa and Monica were helping me move to a beautiful home in Beverly Hills. In between moving stuff around, I slept a lot. I wasn't cranky, just tired. The house was completely empty when we got there, and we put it together in a couple of days. It was crazy! I don't recommend moving while fasting. On the plus side, as I've said, at least my cabinets were empty.

The following year, Lisa flew out and we kidnapped a close friend, Barbara King, to do the cleanse with us. Lisa had never seen *Downton Abbey*, so we decided to watch a couple of seasons during the fast. We spent the day shopping for the cleanse but were in our flannel pajamas at four in the afternoon. While we fasted, we watched two seasons of *Downton Abbey* and old movies like *Joan of Arc*. We barely moved. We had a great time! During the week, Lisa made a big pot of chicken soup and quinoa with veggies.

Barbara wasn't with us 100 percent at first. She was hesitant about doing the cleanse. After 14 days, she felt so amazing that she decided to extend the cleanse for another 14 days. She did the last 2 weeks on her own. The results of her blood work were eye opening. The before test showed high levels of heavy metals like mercury. After 28 days, the elevated levels had returned to normal. She was sold!

We all decided to do the cleanse at least once a year.

REAL TIME CHANGE

The first 2 days were very hard. I recommend that you do the cleanse with a friend. My sister-in-law was very motivating for me.

DALE LAWRENCE
DANVERS, MASSACHUSETTS

ME: To tell you the truth, I never could have done it on my own. My girlfriends kept me in line. It's great to have someone to talk to who is going through the same thing. It's the buddy system.

Thinking of those times reminds me that it's great to do the cleanse with a friend or family member. You can encourage each other and check in with each other about what's happening. The group of women who tried the cleanse while I was writing the book really appreciated the support of a community. If you can't find someone to do the cleanse with you—and even if you do have cleanse buddies—check out my Web site tothefullestbook.com where you can chat with others who are as committed to change as you are, share your experiences, and learn from the tips and recipes they post.

REAL TIME CHANGE

I have one friend who cleanses all of the time, but when I omitted dairy, gluten, booze, and sugar, she couldn't handle it. I stuck to my guns and called her on it!

Some of the people I know aren't the most generous bunch. . . . One friend described me as looking radiant. Another friend said I look "skinny." My husband noticed my weight loss. I think when people see you happy, they may feel threatened—like my anti-cleanse friend who cleanses. Perhaps she could see changes in me she wished to see in herself. I really don't care if others notice or don't. I have done this for myself, and I feel great. Truly, that feeling is beyond satisfying.

MICHELE BLOOM
SOUTH ORANGE, NEW JERSEY

ME: Talk about peer pressure! Don't let people's negativity get to you. You are doing this for yourself. You know how good you feel about the commitment you have made. You must be doing something right if people feel the need to put you down!

PEOPLE'S REACTIONS MIGHT SURPRISE YOU

Everyone will want to know what you are doing. Don't expect everyone to be supportive. Be prepared for some people to say you're crazy, that it's too extreme, that you'll never be able to keep it up. Others will push food and drinks on you. People will ignore you when you try to refuse dessert. "Here, I'm only cutting you a sliver of this flourless chocolate cake. You have to try it," they'll say in spite of your protests. Or "Just have one drink with us to celebrate. Don't be a party pooper."

Don't allow these thoughtless people to undermine your determination. They don't realize how cruel they are being—at least consciously. Ignoring or making light of your efforts is actually disrespectful. Some of your friends and family might just resent you for trying to change. Though they are not willing to make the effort themselves, they fear you will leave them behind after you lose weight and rejuvenate.

REAL TIME CHANGE

I think, overall, people want to be supportive but often are not, without even knowing it. Take, for example, the fact that I love cake. If you know I'm trying to refrain from eating cake, why bring me some? Or when I say, "Thanks, but I'm cutting that out of my diet," they come back with, "Oh, just a little piece then." Or, God forbid, you're out to dinner and don't order an alcoholic beverage. "Oh, come on. Have a drink with us." If you say, "No I better not, I'm driving," you might get, "Oh, one drink is fine—don't be a stick in the mud." It's like peer pressure. They're not trying to sabotage your efforts, but they're not helping. If you're like me, you end up feeling guilty, because what I want to do is throw the cake out after they leave.

ILIANA GUIBERT
NEW YORK, NEW YORK

ME: What happened to respect for another's wishes, desires, commitments? This is so wrong, but it does happen all the time. Like the saying, misery loves company, people want you to join them when they indulge. When you resist, you make them aware of their bad choices. They may not realize that's what's happening, because they convince themselves that you deserve a treat. But you know better.

When your transformation begins, not everyone will be thrilled. For as many people who compliment you on your glow or weight loss, there will be those who are grudging in their comments. "I see you're losing weight—make sure to stop before you look gaunt. Losing too much can be so aging." Or "Honestly, why are you bothering? You know you'll only gain it all back." Or "Right. Everyone's doing cleanses—didn't know you were so trendy." Some people will be cynical and mean-spirited. When they are, don't let it get to you. It is more a reflection of what they think of themselves. They are hopeless and don't think they deserve the best. If they don't, neither do you in their minds. Don't be thrown when people criticize or predict failure. As the quote that opens this book says, "They're telling you their story, not yours."

You are accomplishing something important and have to stay strong. After a short time, you are going to be feeling so good that their negativity and thoughtlessness will bounce right off you, because you'll know that making a commitment to yourself is the best decision you have ever made. You will be sure inside that you are doing the right thing, and they can't stand that you have.

REAL TIME CHANGE

My husband and daughter are big crunch snack fans. I did miss tortilla chips and crunchy snacks, especially when I could hear them crunching. As the days went by, cravings did lessen, but it also became easier to practice Lorraine's mantra of looking the food square in the eye and asking it, "What are you going to do for me?" If the clear answer was "Nothing," I had no problem moving on.

MICHELE BLOOM
SOUTH ORANGE, NEW JERSEY

ME: That really is my mantra! I'm glad you've made it your own. It works. Who needs to eat anything that hurts you rather than gets you to where you want to be—healthy and happy?

COLD TURKEY OR EASE INTO IT?

I was so gung-ho and desperate to jump-start change in my life that I was ready to go cold turkey. Once I make up my mind, there's no holding me back. Some of you might want to jump right in as I did, or you might need to prepare by weaning yourself from foods you will not be eating. If you have a caffeine, sugar, simple carb, or alcohol habit, you might want to withdraw gradually. You should begin cutting back on the foods you will have a hard time giving up a week before you start the cleanse.

Pre-Cleanse Preparation

If you are not ready to go cold turkey, you might want to ease into eliminating foods from your diet. Lisa suggests the following schedule the week before you start the cleanse:

Friday: Reduce the amount of coffee you drink each day until Tuesday, when you stop drinking coffee altogether.

Sunday: Reduce the amount of alcohol you drink until Wednesday, when you stop completely.

Monday: Cut out sugar from your diet. Read labels. Anything containing more than 5 grams of sugar per serving is not for you.

Tuesday: Cut back on gluten until you are down to none on Friday.

Wednesday: Say good-bye to dairy products.

Friday, D-Day: You are free of caffeine, alcohol, sugar, gluten, and dairy and ready for your cleanse.

If you have an especially strong dependence on one food, you might want to make that your priority and start to cut back gradually on that food from Friday to the Friday that you begin the cleanse. Follow the schedule above for the other foods that are disappearing from your diet.

You can do this countdown or dive right in—it's your call. You know what works for you.

You are ready to roll. I'm so excited for you, because you are going to have a life-changing experience. If you are like so many of the women I know, you have tried many fad diets that succeeded for a while, until the old habits returned along with the weight. That is not going to happen this time. We are talking about a fundamental change in your relationship with food and with yourself. You are tapping into your power to shape the way you want to be. Remember to love the struggle!

When you know yourself, you are empowered.
When you accept yourself, you are invincible.
—TINA LIFFORD

7

The 14-Day Liver Cleanse

This chapter is a day-by-day guide to the cleanse, with all you need to know to do the three stages without a glitch. After the first 2 days of fasting, you will find an overview of how to eat to support the cleanse, including what foods to avoid. You will want to reintroduce solid foods strategically and not overwhelm your digestive system as you break the fast. The supplements and meal plans for each day are clearly laid out. We developed the simple menus with practicality in mind. We wanted to make sure you had leftovers that you could recycle in other meals or as snacks. That's how I eat. It's great to have delicious food in the fridge or freezer ready to go. There is also a shopping list of the fresh food you will need for this 2-week period.

Okay! So you are prepared to begin. When Friday morning finally comes, you will initiate making your best vision of yourself a lasting reality.

STAGE 1: DAYS 1 AND 2 (FASTING)

You will not chew during the first 2 days of your liver cleanse. I repeat: No food is eaten for 48 hours. When I heard this, I thought, *No way! I don't know if I can get through 2 days without eating.* But I was determined to take action to clean up my act. I figured I could do anything for 2 days. What surprised me was that I was not hungry at all—and I am an eater! I had visions of myself gnawing on the furniture. Though I expected to be starving, the nutritional supplements actually kept me feeling full. It really wasn't that much of a struggle not to eat.

REAL TIME CHANGE

On the fast—not eating: It's not even the fact that I'm hungry, but more so that I miss eating. Meals are definitely a part of the day I look forward to! At lunchtime I wanted to get my usual salad. Instead, I went out for a walk and did a little window-shopping. That took my mind off of it!

ELIZABETH BLOOM
NEW YORK, NEW YORK

ME: During my fast, I realized how much time I spent thinking and doing food. I wasn't thinking about what I was going to eat next. I had so much more time! Without stopping for meals, you have time to go for a walk around the block and look at things. Take it all in.

I did miss the social aspect of sitting down to have a meal—it's a time to take a break, relax, and enjoy. I organize my day around meals. Not eating freed up a lot of time and energy.

When we started to do the cleanse, Lisa said, "It's like planting a garden. You have to prepare the soil." That's something I know about. Starting a garden is hard work! You have to take a hoe and shovel and turn over the soil, break it up, and get rid of all the weeds, roots, and rocks before you can plant the seeds or young plants. If you want the plants to thrive, the earth has to be made ready. This is the hardest part of making a garden. These two fast days are the hardest part of your transformation into wellness. You have chosen to set the soil to support your own growth. By not eating anything but nutrient-dense shakes and supplements, you are preparing your body to eliminate toxins and to receive real, wholesome food.

REAL TIME CHANGE

After the first two shake-only days, I was committed. Obviously you feel lighter if you don't eat, but that was a good boost for me both physically and psychologically. In the first week, I felt a boost of sorts, but it was more of a mental-commitment kind of boost. A "Hey, Michele, you feel great. Good for you! Keep it up!" kind of boost.

MICHELE BLOOM
SOUTH ORANGE, NEW JERSEY

ME: Isn't it nice to finally do something for yourself? Staying positive and feeling good about yourself is part of the total transformation you are working at.

Look on the bright side—at least you get the hardest part over right away.

Meal Plans for Days 1 and 2

Morning:

Start the day with a glass of filtered water.
2 scoops protein powder mixed with 8 ounces rice or almond milk (believe me, the drink tastes 100 percent better with rice or almond milk than with filtered water)
2 multivitamin/mineral capsules

Evening:

2 scoops protein powder mixed with 8 ounces rice or almond milk
2 multivitamin/mineral capsules

Before bed:

Glass of water
Make sure to drink 6 to 8 glasses of purified water during the day.
Herbal or green tea counts as a fluid. I grew to love licorice mint tea!

REAL TIME CHANGE

On the first night, I made my evening shake, watched a little *Homeland* on Showtime Anytime, got to bed early, and we were on the back stretch with the fasting portion of the plan. Dare I say a piece of cake!!

I did get a little grouchy on the second night—one of the reasons I went to bed so early, to spare my family!

LORETTA LANG STOKES
BEVERLY, MASSACHUSETTS

ME: Bingeing on movies and TV on demand got me through the fast part of the cleanse. I was very tired and hardly got out of bed—when I wasn't running around trying to furnish my new house, something I would not recommend doing! Taking it easy is the best way to begin. Finding a reasonably quiet time to start the cleanse is a big help. Remember that not feeling great the first couple of days is those toxins breaking down.

Don't push yourself during these 2 days as I did the first time I did the cleanse. Take it easy. Skip the Zumba or Spin class. You may be headachy, irritable, and achy, and might break out or feel like you have the flu. Some people have no bad symptoms at all. If you feel bad, remember, the worse you feel, the more toxins are being released. You really needed this cleanse. Drink plenty of water. Get outside and take a walk to get your mind off the fast. Let Mother

REAL TIME CHANGE

The 2-day fast was difficult but manageable. I just reminded myself it was only 2 days and I could do it!! And once the "fog" lifted after Days 4 and 5, I felt so good and clear-headed.

ELIZABETH BLOOM
NEW YORK, NEW YORK

ME: Think of the hard work your body is doing to get rid of all those toxins that have accumulated over time. It amazes me how quickly we bounce back. Cleansing regularly has given me new respect for the body's powerful ability to heal itself. It really is miraculous.

Nature soothe you. And don't forget to take an Epsom salts bath, which will make you feel better and draw out even more toxins through your perspiration. The 2 days will be over before you know it.

Take a Detox Bath Twice a Week to Support the Cleanse

Your skin is an important organ of elimination. Toxins are excreted when you sweat. Relaxing in a hot bath that contains Epsom salts, baking soda, ground ginger, aromatherapy oils, fresh herbs, or any combination of these ingredients at the end of the day is a good way to help your body eliminate toxins. At the same time, your body will absorb the minerals and nutrients you add to the water.

REAL TIME CHANGE

The very first Epsom salts bath I took was revolutionary. I wasn't with my husband or my daughter. I wasn't on my laptop. I wasn't on my phone. I wasn't thinking about work. I was suspended in the tub with nothing but myself. I am someone who enjoys spending time alone, but spending non-task-oriented time with myself was perhaps the biggest gift of this cleanse. I've since spent two spa days with friends. I need to unwind. I need time to merely be. Now I am carving that time out for myself.

MICHELE BLOOM
SOUTH ORANGE, NEW JERSEY

ME: You've learned an important lesson—to unwind. Burning the candle at both ends does not end well. You have to restore yourself regularly if you want to stay healthy. Otherwise, you just wear yourself out. Take time to refresh yourself, and your life will look brighter. Maybe even a nap?

Set aside time for a good soak. Forty minutes is ideal, but plan to spend no fewer than 20 minutes enjoying your bath. Make sure to have a tall glass of water next to the tub—you don't want to get dehydrated.

DETOX BATH

2 cups Epsom salts

1 to 2 cups baking soda

1 tablespoon to ⅓ cup ground ginger (optional)

20 drops aromatherapy oils or fresh herbs (optional)

Explanation of Ingredients

Epsom salts flush out toxins and replenish the level of magnesium in the body, which combats hypertension.

Baking soda has cleansing ability and removes chlorine from the bathwater. Why soak in bathwater that contains toxins? Baking soda will also leave your skin feeling very soft.

Ginger can heat you up, helping to sweat out toxins. It may make your skin turn slightly red for a few minutes, so start slowly with ginger. Work your way up from a tablespoon.

The fragrance of essential oils can make your baths more luxurious. Many oils have therapeutic properties. Tea tree oil or eucalyptus oil are known to help the detoxification process. Lavender or ylang-ylang will be very relaxing. Peppermint is stimulating. Refer to the chart on page 24 to select the right essential oil for your mood. If you choose to try fresh herbs, chamomile is soothing and mint leaves are warming.

Just fill a tub with water as hot as you can stand and stir in the ingredients.

REAL TIME CHANGE

Feeling really good about the completion of Stage 1. Chicken soup simmering on the stove! The house smells amazing. Added some extra veggies. Can't wait to take a bike ride and come back for lunch.

MARY LAMPE SUDDELL
NORTHPORT, NEW YORK

ME: Chicken soup never tasted so good, right? Glad you're moving outside!

You should start sweating in the first few minutes. If you feel too hot, run a little cold water. Remember to drink plenty of water to help flush out the toxins. During your bath, you might like to rub down your body with a dry loofah or brush in long strokes toward your heart to stimulate the lymphatic system, which aids in the release of toxins.

Make sure to get out of the tub carefully. Your body has been working hard, and you might feel a little woozy.

STAGE 2: DAYS 3 TO 7 (ADD FOOD)

You've done it! You have completed the fast part of the cleanse. It wasn't that terrible, was it? That's as bad as it gets. Now you can start to eat again, but you won't be breaking your fast by chowing down on pizza or a cheeseburger and fries. Why would you want to weigh yourself down with heavy, greasy food? This is where the lifestyle change begins to happen. You are going to start making healthy choices that will help your body to detoxify. This diet plan reduces the load of incoming toxins and will improve your body's ability to eliminate toxins that have been stored over time, particularly around your middle. Eating this way will reduce inflammatory stress on your digestive tract, and that allows the intestinal lining to do its job. When toxins and undigested proteins leak from the intestines into the bloodstream, food allergies and sensitivities can develop. The foods at the root of the most common food allergies and sensitivities are:

- Wheat
- Dairy
- Soy
- Eggs
- Seafood
- Nuts (If you know you do not have nut allergies, just avoid peanuts, which are legumes, not nuts.)

Your diet for the rest of the cleanse—the next 12 days—is hypoallergenic, designed to help you identify and minimize the consumption of foods that can cause food allergies and sensitivities. So you will not be eating wheat and gluten-containing grains, dairy, soy, eggs, or seafood. The recommended foods will reduce the stress hormone response, which causes inflammation, and will improve your immune system. This cleanse will give your entire GI system a chance to heal.

Eating clean is an important part of your transformation. The foods in this diet plan decrease your exposure to pesticides, herbicides, artificial colors and flavors, antibiotics, hormones, and preservatives, which are present in abundance in processed food and conventionally farmed produce, poultry, and other livestock. All these additives make your detoxification system work overtime. You have to commit to eating organic fruits and vegetables and free-range, antibiotic-free, and hormone-free poultry and meats if you want the cleanse to be as effective as possible.

Eating to Support Your Liver Cleanse

Foods That Boost Detoxification

Fruits: Avocados, raspberries, strawberries, blueberries, 100% berry juices, bananas, apples, pomegranates, any other organic fresh or frozen fruit except grapes

Vegetables: Broccoli, cabbage, cauliflower, Brussels sprouts, green beans, watercress, arugula, spinach, kale, Swiss chard, collard greens, peppers, celery, cucumbers, bok choy, radishes, turnips, beans and lentils, garlic, onions

Grains: Whole grain brown rice, buckwheat, millet, amaranth, quinoa

Nuts and seeds: Almonds, cashews, walnuts, chia seeds, sunflower seeds, sesame seeds, pumpkin seeds

Dairy: Use a milk substitute like rice or almond milk

Meat: Organic, free-range chicken, organic beef

Fats: Extra virgin olive oil, flaxseed oil, raw virgin coconut oil, grapeseed oil, and other nut and seed oils except for peanut

Drinks: Filtered or bottled water, 100% fruit or vegetable juice, organic herbal tea, organic green tea

Spices and sauces: Celtic sea salt, fresh and dried spices and herbs, garlic

Foods to Avoid on the Cleanse

Fruits: Canned fruit packaged in syrup, high sugar or artificial berry juices, oranges, grapefruit

Vegetables: Corn, canned vegetables in sauces, soybean and soy-based foods, white potatoes

Grains: Refined flours, gluten-containing grains such as wheat, spelt, kamut, rye, oats, and barley

Nuts and seeds: Peanuts (which are actually legumes), soy nuts

Dairy: Milk, cheese, ice cream, yogurt, all dairy-based products

Fats: Margarine, butter, hydrogenated oils, cooking sprays, mayonnaise

Drinks: Coffee, sweetened beverages, alcohol, high sugar or artificially flavored juices, black tea

Spices and sauces: Soy sauce, barbecue sauce, ketchup, relishes

Other: Eggs, fish and shellfish, nonorganic meats, fried foods, artificial flavors, colors, preservatives (especially MSG), sugar, maple syrup, molasses, honey

If you have joint pain, you should consider avoiding foods derived from the nightshade family of plants, including tomatoes, white potatoes, eggplant, peppers of all kinds (except black pepper), paprika, and cayenne.

Celtic Sea Salt

I've noticed so many new salts on the shelves besides standard table salt: pink Himalayan salt, Dead Sea salt, Red Hawaiian sea salt, finishing salt. One is better than the rest: Celtic sea salt, also known as *sel gris* or *fleur de sel*. Commercial salt is very harsh and can be iodized. You do need iodine for your thyroid to work well, but you get enough if you eat a varied diet. An excess of iodine will mess with your metabolism. You should use Celtic sea salt for its many benefits. This naturally moist salt is harvested from the Atlantic seawater off the coast of Brittany, France. The Celtic method of wooden rakes is used to harvest the salt, so that no metal touches the salt. It is then naturally air- and sun-dried in clay ponds and gathered with wooden tools to preserve its living enzymes.

Since it is unrefined, the salt contains all of the 84 beneficial live elements found in seawater, with no chemicals or preservatives or any other additives.

Among the live minerals and trace elements found in Celtic sea salt are iodine, iron, calcium, magnesium, manganese, potassium, and zinc. The appropriate magnesium content ensures that unused sodium is quickly and completely eliminated from the body through the kidneys to prevent harm, which means it does not affect blood pressure. Finally, the best thing about Celtic sea salt is that it brings out the flavor of food.

REAL TIME CHANGE

I thought the Celtic sea salt was magical. I have used other sea salts, but this one is special. The first time I used it, I could tell it was so different, actually enhancing the flavor of food rather than just imparting a saline taste. I am officially a salt snob.

DIANE ARPINO
RAMSEY, NEW JERSEY

ME: Celtic sea salt actually brings out the flavor of food rather than masking it. Lisa and I always say the two things we'd want to have on a desert island would be Celtic sea salt and extra virgin olive oil.

Substitute Warm/Hot Lemon Water for Coffee

A great way to start any day is to drink a cup of warm/hot lemon water when you get up, but it is particularly important when you are on the cleanse for reasons I'll get to. Just squeeze half a lemon into a glass of warm or hot purified water. I like to add a dash of cayenne for a bit of a kick and sometimes just a drop of honey. You won't believe the benefits of drinking hot lemon water. It beats drinking coffee hands down. This simple drink has physical benefits that will help you to get where you want to be:

- **Aids digestion.** Lemon juice helps to flush out toxins, particularly from the digestive tract. Its composition is similar to the acids in saliva and digestive juices. It stimulates the liver to produce bile.
- **Acts as a diuretic.** The increase in the rate of urination helps to eliminate toxins from the body and gets rid of bloat.
- **Boosts your immunity.** The high vitamin C content has anti-inflammatory effects, and high levels of potassium boost nerve and brain function.

REAL TIME CHANGE

Not sure how long it takes to make or break a habit, but I have abandoned my morning cup of coffee for a cup of hot water/half lemon. I have really come to enjoy that and feel no need to go back to a cup of coffee. Small steps . . .

LORETTA LANG STOKES
BEVERLY, MASSACHUSETTS

ME: You've done something I haven't managed to do yet. I haven't been able to give up my morning coffee. Pick your poison, I guess.

- **Balances pH levels.** Lemons are one of the most alkalizing foods for the body. Drinking lemon water regularly can reduce acidity, including uric acid in the joints, one of the primary causes of pain and inflammation.

- **Clears skin.** Vitamin C and other antioxidants fight skin aging, decreasing wrinkles and blemishes. It rejuvenates the skin from the inside out. The alkaline nature of lemon juice kills some of the bacteria that cause acne.

- **Enhances your mood and boosts your energy.** The scent of lemon has mood-enhancing and mind-clearing properties. It can reduce anxiety and depression.

- **Promotes healing.** The vitamin C (ascorbic acid) found in lemons promotes healing and helps to maintain healthy bones, connective tissue, and cartilage.

- **Freshens breath.** You know how crisp and clean lemon juice smells. A warning: Citric acid can erode tooth enamel. It is a good idea to rinse your mouth with purified water after drinking lemon water.

- **Aids in weight loss.** People who maintain a more alkaline diet lose weight faster. Since lemons help to make the body more alkaline, drinking lemon water is a good weight loss aid. Lemons are also high in pectin fiber, which helps fight hunger cravings.

A Little Seed That Packs a Punch

Chia seeds are a superfood. Yep, they are the same seeds that grow into the green hair of Chia Pets. Those little seeds deliver maximal nutrients with minimal

A Guide to Eating on Days 3 to 14 of the Cleanse

Follow these rules for a successful cleanse and for healthy eating for the rest of your life:

- Avoid packaged, prepared, or processed foods, which are filled with toxins and too much salt, sugar, and fat.
- Stick to whole, fresh foods.
- Eat organic fruits and vegetables.
- Don't eat salads until the full 14-day cleanse is complete. You want to give your digestive system a rest. Only eat dark leafy greens like arugula, spinach, and watercress.
- Eat free-range chickens and grass-fed beef that are free of antibiotics and hormones.
- Drink only bottled or filtered water. Aim for six to eight 8-ounce glasses (48 to 64 ounces) a day. Drinking enough water is key to flushing out the toxins from your body. Avoid distilled water, because it lacks minerals.
- Stay away from coffee, soda, alcohol, fruit juices, and black tea.
- Have a healthy snack midmorning and midafternoon to keep your blood sugar level steady.
- Do not eat dinner until you have had your protein shake and supplements. You will be less hungry after you drink your shake.
- Do not be tempted to eat any of the foods on the "Foods to Avoid on the Cleanse" list, because they have the potential to cause inflammation from an allergy or sensitivity. That would strain your liver and your digestive system.
- If you are still a smoker, try to minimize your nicotine exposure. Cut tobacco use by 50 percent during the detox. Better yet, plan to stop entirely.
- After the initial 2 days, you should aim for 1,300 calories per day. This caloric intake will help you to maintain blood sugar without putting a burden on your digestive system.

calories. Chia seeds come from a desert plant that is a member of the mint family and grows in Central America. The seeds were a staple in the diet of the ancient Aztecs and used by Native Americans in the Southwest. These tiny seeds will do a lot for you:

- They are composed of 60 percent omega-3 fatty acids, which makes them one of the richest plant-based sources of omega-3s. The fatty acids in chia seeds can help reduce inflammation and high cholesterol and make you sharper.
- Just 2 tablespoons of chia seeds have 10 grams of fiber, one-third the daily recommended intake of fiber.
- Chia seeds are packed with antioxidants that protect the body from free radicals, aging, and cancer. The antioxidants give them a long shelf life. They last almost 2 years without refrigeration.
- Chia seeds are rich in minerals. Two tablespoons of the seeds contain 18 percent of the daily recommended calcium, 35 percent of phosphorus, 24 percent of magnesium, and 50 percent of manganese. These minerals prevent high blood pressure and help maintain healthy weight, because they are important for burning energy.
- Chia seeds fill you up. The combination of fatty acids, fiber, and the gelling action of chia seeds when mixed with liquids will curb your food cravings.

You can sprinkle chia seeds on vegetables, salads, brown rice, quinoa, and gluten-free oatmeal. Make a habit of using chia the way you do salt. The seeds add a nice crunch when mixed with dry food. After the cleanse, I put a teaspoon of ground chia seeds in my protein shakes to fill me up. When wet, chia becomes like tapioca. There are great recipes for vanilla and chocolate chia puddings on pages 221 and 222, which you can eat during the cleanse.

You Can Eat Again!

Now that you've returned to the world of solid food, we want to give you some guidance on how to reintroduce food after your fast. We suggest meal plans for what to eat for the remaining 12 days of the cleanse. These foods will gently ease you back into eating solid food again. If you find that you are not very hungry after your dinner shake, do not force yourself to eat. I often found that I didn't want very much for dinner. If you are starving in the middle of the day, you might want to switch out the heavier dinner menu with the lunch menu. I did it all the time. You are not supposed to be hungry while you are on the cleanse. I couldn't have done it otherwise. The idea is to eat well, not to deprive yourself.

The menus are intentionally varied to show you that hunger is not part of the program and that eating clean has endless flavorful options. Let's face it, we are all busy and want to be able to eat healthy food without spending hours in the kitchen. For me, simple food is the answer. **The simpler the food, the cleaner it is.**

REAL TIME CHANGE

I thought it would be really difficult. Once I got into a routine, I was amazed at myself. I have always been a carb addict, but this cleanse and the Clean Up Your Act Diet showed me I can eat good, healthy food and feel satisfied. Most important, I felt good after I ate. When I was carbed out, I felt sluggish and, frankly, unhealthy.

ANA NAPOLES
BLOOMFIELD, NEW JERSEY

ME: We are what we eat. When we eat fresh food that's alive, we feel vibrant. When we load ourselves down with sugar and simple carbs, we feel heavy and dead.

I have to confess that I tend to eat the same things every day. Then I don't have to think about it. For example, I have go-to snacks. I eat an entire box of blueberries or raspberries in an afternoon! I love Justin's Almond Butter. A tablespoon on a rice cake is everything a snack should be. I make a big batch of my own basic hummus and add an assortment of ingredients for extra flavor, depending on my mood. I roast Brussels sprouts, broccoli, cauliflower, parsnips, carrots, or kale until they are crispy and munch on them like chips. Soups are a great option—a big pot goes a long way. I freeze the soup in small portions, but I've been known to have soup every day of the week. I keep cooked quinoa and grilled or poached boneless chicken breasts in the fridge and the freezer to use as a base for a side dish or meal. A grilled, poached, or roasted protein with a steamed or roasted vegetable is my fallback dinner. I use a grill pan and a wok, which make preparing a meal quick and easy. You can find recipes for some of the meals on the cleanse starting on page 181.

As you make conscious choices about eating what is good for you, make mental notes of how you feel after eating or drinking something. Acknowledge how eating clean makes you feel compared to wolfing down a big bowl of pasta or a sweet dessert. You start to realize that how you have been feeling has a lot to do with what you've been eating. Eating food that is fresh and alive will lift you up and make you glow.

REAL TIME CHANGE

I am both excited and nervous about the next phase. I am excited because now eating any of the forbiddens would be a deliberate choice, as I don't crave dairy, gluten products, alcohol, sugar, or soy. I know that eggs hurt my stomach and am coming to understand that nightshades are hard for me, too. I feel alert and awake, energized and clear.

MICHELE BLOOM
SOUTH ORANGE, NEW JERSEY

ME: It's great to know what foods your body is sensitive to so that you can steer clear. Knowing if your body reacts badly to certain foods makes it easier to do without them. It's all about making conscious food choices.

Just Because It's Healthy
Doesn't Mean You Can Eat All You Want

A good friend has been ill. I visited her with a huge basket of healthy food to help her get back on her feet. She was not doing a cleanse, so I included some of my favorite gluten-free cookies. When I called a couple of days later to check in, she said, "I don't know, Lorraine. I ate all those cookies, and I didn't feel so great." Even if what you are eating is healthy, the amount you consume of some foods has to be limited.

Portion control is a big part of changing your relationship with the food you eat, and we have become too used to supersized portions. Here are some basic guidelines for eyeballing how much you are eating:

- 1 cup = a baseball
- ½ cup = a lightbulb
- 1 ounce or 2 tablespoons = a golf ball
- 1 tablespoon = a poker chip
- 3 ounces of chicken or meat = a deck of cards
- 4 ounces of chicken or meat = two eggs
- 3 ounces of fish = a checkbook
- 4 ounces of fish = two eggs

It's easy to sit with a bowl of nuts and eat the whole thing or to slather a rice cake with a ton of almond butter. You have to be aware of how much you are eating. These are reasonable portions.

- Almonds, walnuts, pumpkin seeds: ¼ cup—about a handful, which is 23 almonds
- Raw cashews: 10
- Cooked quinoa, brown rice, gluten-free pasta: ½ cup as a side dish, 1 cup as a main course
- Nut butters: 1 tablespoon
- Extra virgin olive oil: 2 tablespoons
- Cheese (feta is on the menu after the cleanse): 1 ounce = two dice
- Sweet potato (after cleanse): 3 ounces = computer mouse
- Apples: 4 ounces = the size of a baseball
- Fruit consumption: three servings a day
- Sugary fruits like grapes: avoid them (they're sugar bombs)
- Pineapple: ½ cup a day
- One banana a day
- As many vegetables, melons, and berries as you want

The key is to learn to know when you have had enough to eat, when you are no longer hungry. You have to be able to push away from the table before you are stuffed. It's good to be a little bit hungry after a meal rather uncomfortably full. There's a difference between being stuffed and feeling satisfied. As you follow the Clean Up Your Act Plan, you'll see that it does not take that much to fill you up.

REAL TIME CHANGE

Going food shopping was not the best thing to do hungry. I bought every-thing . . . but I realized how I eat unconsciously . . . a bite of this or that, a sample at a store. It did not take a lot of effort to walk past the free sam-ples or to think about not having something even if I thought I wanted to at that moment.

LUCILLE IRCHA
NEW YORK, NEW YORK

ME: Supermarkets can be dangerous if you're hungry! If you stay on the outside walls, you'll avoid some of the worst temptations. And fill your basket with fresh food. It's great that shopping made you aware of mind-less eating—those samples get me every time!

Shopping List for Days 3 to 7

If you have the energy, go shopping on the second day of your fast for the food you will eat from Days 3 to 7. It will take your mind off the fast. Feel free to be creative with the vegetables, herbs, and spices you use. Here is what you will need if you follow the meal plans.

Apples	Chicken, whole (4½ to 5 pounds)
Avocados	Chopped beef
Basil	Eggplant
Bell peppers, red and yellow	Frozen organic fruit for shake
Blueberries	Garlic
Brussels sprouts	Green beans
Cantaloupe	Hummus (ready-made if you do not
Carrots	want to make your own)
Cayenne pepper	Kale
Celery	Lemons
Cherry tomatoes	Lentils
Chicken breasts	Onions, red and yellow

(continued)

Parsley	Spaghetti squash
Pumpkin seeds	Spinach
Radishes	Steak
Raspberries	Veggie burger
Sesame seeds	Zucchini

Look over the meal plans before you go shopping. You might want to change a menu or snack on something different. Make this cleanse your own, because you won't stop eating this way when the 2 weeks are over. As long as you follow the dos and don'ts—and stay away from sugar, gluten, and dairy—you make the decisions about what's right for you.

Most people start to feel different during this stage of the cleanse. Your body is working hard to release the toxins stored in your fat cells. Since you are eating clean food that will not bog you down by adding to your toxic load, you will start to feel change. Many people feel lighter, more centered, less bloated, and more energetic. I know I did about Day 5. This hint of improvement is so encouraging that you will not have trouble sticking with the program.

Supplements for Days 3 to 7

You will be adding four phytonutrient capsules a day to your supplement regimen.

Morning:

2 scoops protein powder mixed with 8 ounces rice or almond milk; blend in berries, pears, peaches, or other fruit for extra flavor (I buy big bags of frozen organic fruit, because a cold shake is delicious)
2 multivitamin/mineral capsules
2 phytonutrient capsules

Evening:

2 scoops protein powder mixed with 8 ounces rice or almond milk and fruit of choice, if desired
2 multivitamin/mineral capsules
2 phytonutrient capsules

Meal Plans for Days 3 to 7

DAY 3

The day after your fast, you should eat lightly. A homemade chicken soup is the way to go. In fact, you should always have some in your freezer.

On rising:

Hot lemon water

Breakfast:

Protein shake

Supplements

Midmorning snack:

Almond butter on apple slices

Water or tea

Lunch:

Simple Chicken Soup (page 189)—steamed veggies and quinoa can be added

Iced tea with lemon or water

Snack:

Pumpkin seeds

Dinner:

Important: Be sure to drink your protein shake and take your supplements before you eat. If you wait a bit to eat, you might find you are not that hungry. I drank my protein shake before I started to get dinner together. It reduced my appetite, leaving me with leftovers for the next day.

Protein shake

Supplements

Simple Chicken Soup

Water or tea

If you are hungry at any time during the day, feel free to have soup or tea.

Before bed:

Glass of water

Make sure to have a total of 6 to 8 glasses of liquid a day. Tea counts.

DAY 4

On rising:
Hot lemon water

Breakfast:
Protein shake
Supplements

Midmorning snack:
Raw cashews
Water or tea

Lunch:
Vegetable Quinoa (page 213)
Water or tea

Midafternoon snack:
Fresh blueberries
Water or tea

Dinner:
Protein shake
Supplements
Hamburger with guacamole or avocado slices—no bun
Water or tea

Before bed:
Glass of water

DAY 5

On rising:
Hot lemon water

Breakfast:
Protein shake
Supplements

Midmorning snack:
Almond butter on rice cake
Water or tea

Lunch:

Hummus with celery, carrots, and radishes (see recipes on page 185 for basic hummus and varieties, or choose an organic ready-made brand)

Water or tea

Dinner:

Protein shake

Supplements

Grilled chicken breast or paillard and roasted Brussels sprouts (see recipe for Roasted Veggies on page 212; make extra Brussels sprouts for snacks)

Water or tea

Before bed:

Glass of water

DAY 6

On rising:

Hot lemon water

Breakfast:

Protein shake

Supplements

Midmorning snack:

Cantaloupe chunks

Water or tea

Lunch:

Hot Lentil Salad (page 214)

Water or tea

Midafternoon Snack:

Roasted Brussels sprouts

Water or tea

Dinner:

Protein shake

Supplements

Spaghetti squash with Quick Cherry Tomato Sauce (page 197)

Water or tea

Before bed:

Glass of water

DAY 7

On rising:

Hot lemon water

Breakfast:

Protein shake

Supplements

Midmorning snack:

Raw almonds

Lunch:

Veggie Burger (see recipes starting on page 201) with kale chips (see suggestion in the Roasted Veggies recipe page 212); make extra kale chips for snacking. If you buy prepared veggie burgers, make sure soy and corn are not on the ingredient list. They often sneak in.

Midafternoon snack:

Raspberries

Water or tea

REAL TIME CHANGE

I know it's only been almost a week, but I'm down 5 pounds and my clothes are already feeling differently. Eating clean has never felt so good or so easy, except for the first 2 days, of course. Feeling happy and energized.

MARY LAMPE SUDDELL
NORTHPORT, NEW YORK

ME: When you see and feel the change in you, it's not hard to follow the plan. I just wanted to feel better and better, and didn't want to go back to the way I used to feel. And there's nothing like when other people see it in you. You've got to love that!

Dinner:

Protein shake

Supplements

Grilled or broiled steak and steamed spinach with sesame seeds

Water or tea

Before bed:

Glass of water

STAGE 3: DAYS 8 TO 14

Your body is now transitioning into the second phase of liver detoxification. The fat-soluble toxins released in Stage 1 are being converted to water-soluble compounds and eliminated. Now you are really going to feel a change as you flush those toxins out of your body. Be sure to drink a lot of water to speed the process. I found at this point that I didn't really miss eating all the things I had given up. I was losing weight steadily and just felt healthier. My aches and pains started to go away. My sleep improved so much I was springing out of bed in the morning. During this stage, you'll see a payoff for all your hard work.

Supplements for Days 8 to 14

You will add two more phytonutrients a day, for a total of three in the morning and three in the evening. This is what you will be taking to support Days 8 to 14 of your cleanse:

Morning:

2 scoops protein powder mixed with 8 ounces rice or almond milk and fruit of choice, if desired

2 multivitamin/mineral capsules

3 phytonutrient capsules

Evening:

2 scoops protein powder mixed with 8 ounces rice or almond milk and fruit of choice, if desired

2 multivitamin/mineral capsules

3 phytonutrient capsules

REAL TIME CHANGE

The first few days of the cleanse, maybe my body was a little shocked—a welcomed surprise.

Second week: The first days were good, because you're excited and pumped, and then it gets hard to maintain, but then you have to start up again, get back on track. Don't be a runaway train.

It did get easier, then I'd have a day here and there that were tougher, but overall it got easier. On the not-so-easy day, I just had to stay strong and tell myself not to let one tough day turn into three or four.

ILIANA MCGINNIS
NEW YORK, NEW YORK

ME: Not being too hard on yourself is smart. Loving the struggle is what it's all about. When you accept that it takes effort to change, you can pump up your determination to stay on track.

Shopping List for Days 8 to 14

These are the foods you will need if you follow the meal plans. Check the recipes to get a sense of how much to buy.

Asparagus	Cumin
Avocados	Garlic
Bananas	Green beans
Basil	Hummus
Broccoli	Kale
Cabbage	Leeks
Carrots	Lemons
Celery	Lime
Chicken	Mangoes
Chili powder	Mixed berries
Chopped beef or turkey	Nectarines
Cilantro	Onions, red and yellow
Collard greens	Parsnips

Peaches

Pears

Peppers

Pineapple

Plums

Roast beef, thinly sliced

Tomatoes

Turkey, thinly sliced

White mushrooms

Meal Plans for Days 8 to 14

DAY 8

On rising:

Hot lemon water

Breakfast:

Protein shake

Supplements

Midmorning snack:

Mixed nuts: almonds, cashews, and walnuts

Lunch:

Simple Chicken Soup (page 189) with Vegetable Quinoa (page 213)

Water or tea

Midafternoon snack:

Kale chips

Water or tea

Dinner:

Protein shake

Supplements

Chicken-broccoli-pepper-onion stir-fry with $\frac{1}{2}$ cup quinoa, brown rice, or gluten-free long-grain rice

Water or tea

Before bed:

Glass of water

DAY 9

On rising:

Hot lemon water

Breakfast:

Protein shake

Supplements

Midmorning snack:

Almond butter on celery

Water or tea

Lunch:

Mushroom Pâté (page 187) on rice cakes

Water or tea

Midafternoon snack:

Sliced tomato with fresh basil and extra virgin olive oil

Water or tea

Dinner:

Protein shake

Supplements

Turkey or beef chili with kidney beans on ½ cup quinoa

Water or iced tea

Before bed:

Glass of water

REAL TIME CHANGE

Days 6–14: Once I got into the swing of things and knew what I could and could not eat, it got easier. Plus when you start to feel better and reap the benefits of the cleanse, it keeps you motivated.

LORETTA LANG STOKES
BEVERLY, MASSACHUSETTS

ME: Eating clean has become automatic for me. When I do stray, I feel it. It makes me question if it's worth it!

DAY 10

On rising:

Hot lemon water

Breakfast:

Protein shake

Supplements

Midmorning snack:

Pineapple

Lunch:

Quinoa with olive oil, garlic, and capers (I love this and eat it all the time—easy and delicious)

Water or tea

Midafternoon snack:

Hummus with carrots and celery

Dinner:

Protein shake

Supplements

Black Bean Soup (page 190) with guacamole on top, or Multitasking Vegetable Soup (page 191)

Water or tea

Before bed:

Glass of water

DAY 11

On rising:

Hot lemon water

Breakfast:

Protein shake

Supplements

Midmorning snack:

Almond butter on pear slices

Water or tea

Lunch:

Turkey or beef chili leftovers

Water or tea

Midafternoon snack:

Sliced avocado with paprika

Water or tea

Dinner:

Protein shake

Supplements

Roasted Lemon Chicken (page 193) with steamed asparagus
(make extra asparagus)

Water or tea

Before bed:

Glass of water

REAL TIME CHANGE

There were alternating days during the 2 weeks when my energy was boundless, then days where it felt as though I was dragging a large ball and chain around all day. At the end of the cleanse, the ball and chain were gone . . . the energy I needed to get through my day came more easily without struggle.

DIANE ARPINO
RAMSEY, NEW JERSEY

ME: Say good-bye to that ball and chain! You don't need anything to hold you back.

DAY 12

On rising:

Hot lemon water

Breakfast:

Protein shake

Supplements

Midmorning snack:
Hummus with carrots and celery

Lunch:
Thin-sliced roast beef or turkey wrapped around
cooked asparagus

Midafternoon snack:
Vanilla Chia Seed Pudding (page 220)
Water or tea

Dinner:
Protein shake
Supplements
Stuffed Peppers (page 195); make extra for leftovers

Before bed:
Glass of water

DAY 13

On rising:
Hot lemon water

Breakfast:
Protein shake
Supplements

Midmorning snack:
Almond butter on banana slices
Water or tea

Lunch:
Leftover cold sliced chicken with steamed vegetables
Water or tea

Midafternoon snack:
Peach slices, nectarines, or plums with balsamic vinegar
and mint
Water or tea

Dinner:

Protein shake

Supplements

Grilled chicken breast with Mango Salsa (page 186) and steamed green beans with almonds

Water or tea

Before bed:

Glass of water

DAY 14

On rising:

Hot lemon water

Breakfast:

Protein shake

Supplements

Midmorning snack:

Mixed nuts

Lunch:

Black Bean or Multitasking Vegetable Soups (pages 190, 191)

Water or tea

REAL TIME CHANGE

I'm on my feet all day, and I'd been feeling it. The backaches, body aches, and the bad pain in my left foot are gone. I no longer get charley horses, and most of all, my constipation is gone. I sleep great!

WENDY NAPOLES
NUTLEY, NEW JERSEY

ME: Being pain free is liberating, isn't it? There is no reason to suffer in silence and to accept those aches and pains as inevitable. If you take care of your body, it will take care of you.

Midafternoon snack:

Mushroom Pâté (page 187) with fresh carrots and celery

Dinner:

Protein shake

Supplements

Steak with baked carrot and parsnip fries sprinkled with a little cumin

Water or tea

Before bed:

Glass of water

REAL TIME CHANGE

While still on shakes and supplements, I didn't really crave anything. I was tempted by smells. I did crave stew, but that's a shift from craving Cheetos. Yesterday, I was craving chicken. The day before that I was craving fresh fruit. Go figure!

MICHELE BLOOM
SOUTH ORANGE, NEW JERSEY

ME: Your body is speaking to you! It's great when your food addictions disappear.

I want you to take your arm, wrap it around your neck, and give yourself a pat on the back. You have completed the cleanse. You've already seen how dropping dairy, sugar, and gluten has affected you in just 2 weeks. Don't you look fresher and feel less bloated? How is your energy? Your mood? I'm sure you're riding high after completing the 14-day cleanse. You have taken control of your life, and nothing feels better. If you can do that with what you eat, you have the power to transform your life. It's a miracle—the biggest gift of all.

Now the rest of this journey is really up to you. You have the tools, so you just need to apply them consciously every day. Eating clean will become second nature to you, if it hasn't already. You have made an incredible change in your life very quickly. Have your tastebuds changed? Do you have the same cravings? I have to let you know that it just gets better. Keep up the good fight!

In the next chapter, the Clean Up Your Act Diet will show you how to continue making clean eating a way of life. We've expanded the list of go-to foods and included healthy and delicious substitutes for ingredients that are not on the plan, as well as ideas for quick, tasty meals and snacks. We give you guidelines for how to eat for the rest of your life. Be proud of what you've accomplished and continue on the path to vibrant health.

Life has no remote. Get up and change it yourself.
—AUTHOR UNKNOWN

8

The Clean Up Your Act Diet—The Way to Eat for the Rest of Your Life

You've finished your 2-week cleanse. Don't you feel cleaner and lighter? Your body will continue to change inside. Your commitment to yourself doesn't stop after 14 days. As long as you keep eating clean, you will feel better and better. When I finished my first cleanse, I asked Lisa, "So now what?" She asked where I wanted to be in a year. I got what she was saying. It doesn't end with the cleanse. My goals had to be long term. Once I achieved them, there would be new ones. That's what I mean by being a work in progress.

This is not about two weeks of following a plan and then back to your old ways. You have to have your own self-improvement plan that you attack one step at a time. I had a weight goal that took me a year to reach. I don't weigh myself every day. I can tell how I'm doing by how my clothes fit. I've been able to keep

131

the weight off and can fit into pants that I couldn't get up past my thighs before I cleaned up my act. I also wanted to be great in my work. I'm having a wonderful time playing Angela on *Rizzoli & Isles*. I wanted to appreciate the little things every day—all the way down to a single blade of grass. Working on that has enriched my life. If you want to get yourself back, slow and steady wins the race. You have to make clean eating a way of life, so that your body can heal itself and find its true balance.

REAL TIME CHANGE

I don't think I can completely change my eating habits in 30 days. I've had these bad/poor eating habits my entire life, but I've started to chip away at it.

ILIANA GUIBERT
NEW YORK, NEW YORK

ME: Remember, slow and steady wins the race. It's only a matter of time until you have nothing to do with bad eating.

The Clean Up Your Act Diet is a simple way to eat that will keep you in great shape. In the past 2 weeks, you have started to think differently about food. The benefits of eating this way are probably visible at this point, not to mention how you feel. Those changes should give you the incentive to make this diet a way of life.

The goal remains to eat fresh, organic food without gluten, sugar, and dairy. If you eat clean and watch your portions, you will shed unwanted pounds, but more important, you will wipe out chronic physical complaints for good and prevent problems from developing. When you first thought about eating gluten free, sugar free, and dairy free, it probably seemed too tough, even for 14 days. It did to me—and here I am, 4 years and counting. I don't even remember what it was like to eat the way I did before, but I have vivid memories of how I felt. Knowing how great I feel now, there is no way I'm ever going back. I hope the physical, mental, and spiritual changes you've seen while doing the cleanse will convince you that eating clean can have a powerful effect on your life. The good news is that now you can eat a broader range of food.

REAL TIME CHANGE

I became better at listening to my belly and not my tastebuds. As a result of the cleanse, my whole mind-set has changed as have my cravings. While I always ate nutrition-rich food, I also stuffed myself with sugar, caffeine, and dairy. Now, without sugar, caffeine, dairy, and gluten, it seems my whole constitution has changed. I crave a nectarine or hummus with veggies. I don't miss sugar or sugary snacks.

ELIZABETH BLOOM
NEW YORK, NEW YORK

ME: Well, you don't miss them, because there's nothing there for you.

FOODS YOU CAN ADD TO YOUR DIET

Having completed the cleanse, you can reintroduce foods to your diet that will increase your choices exponentially. I never thought I would crave salad, but by the time I finish my cleanse, a salad seems like a major treat!

- Coffee, one cup daily (hurray!)
- Stevia
- Eggs, organic, free-range
- Egg whites
- Lamb
- Salads
- Low-mercury fish and seafood (see list on page 137), no more than two servings a week
- Goat milk, yogurt, cheese
- Sheep milk, yogurt, cheese
- Sweet potatoes
- Gluten-free oatmeal
- Gluten-free cream of quinoa
- Gluten-free cream of rice

- Gluten-free pasta (I love the quinoa pastas. I keep it to no more than twice a week, and I watch the size of my portion.)
- Gluten-free wraps
- Rice wraps

Adding these foods will give you a much greater range in meal planning. Eggs alone are so versatile. Now, you will be able to take clean eating to another level.

REAL TIME CHANGE

The foods in the clean eating plan are delicious and satisfying. I never felt completely famished or wanting more. And it was fun working in some new foods to my diet—like quinoa, which is just so yummy with vegetables.

ELIZABETH BLOOM
NEW YORK, NEW YORK

ME: I have grown to love quinoa—I even eat it for breakfast with blueberries and maple syrup. I always have cooked quinoa in my refrigerator and freezer. I use it as a base for salads, but I also toss some in green salads and soup. Quinoa has replaced pasta in my life, and that's a big job!

Organic or Not?

During the cleanse, it was important to eat organic everything, because you were giving your liver a rest. Now that you're clean, it's always smart to continue to eat organic food. Your toxic load will quickly build up again if you eat food raised with harmful chemicals. Since you are exposed to so many toxins already, you don't want to add to your toxic load by eating commercially raised meat and produce. Sometimes you might have trouble finding the organic vegetables you want, or the expense might be a problem. This rule can be bent a bit.

Buying locally raised produce, eggs, poultry, and meat is always a good choice. The food is fresher, because it hasn't had to travel far. Much local food is produced on a small scale, which usually cuts out the worst practices of commercial farming. I like to know the chickens whose eggs I eat. Eating produce in season—cycling through the crops as they are harvested—is a great rhythm to get into. One of the things I love about Los Angeles is that everything is in season all the time. The farmers' markets there are beautiful, so colorful and abundant. It's easy to eat clean there all year, and it's so much part of the culture.

If for one reason or another, eating 100 percent organic is not for you, there is a way to pick and choose the conventionally grown fruits and vegetables with the lowest pesticide load and to avoid the produce with the highest. Every year, the Environmental Working Group produces a list of the safest conventionally grown crops along with a list of the foods you should always buy organic, which they call the "Clean Fifteen" and the "Dirty Dozen." Here are the 2014 winners and losers:

The Clean Fifteen

Since these fruits and vegetables have the lowest pesticide loads, you do not have to buy them organic.

Avocados	Papayas
Sweet corn	Kiwi
Pineapples	Eggplant
Cabbage	Grapefruit
Sweet peas (frozen)	Cantaloupe (domestic)
Onions	Cauliflower
Asparagus	Sweet potatoes
Mangoes	

The Dirty Dozen

The foods on the following list had the highest pesticide load, making them the most important to buy organic.

Apples	Peaches
Strawberries	Spinach
Grapes	Sweet bell peppers
Celery	Nectarines (imported)

Cucumbers

Snap peas (imported)

Cherry tomatoes

Potatoes

Plus these foods, which may contain very toxic insecticides:

Hot peppers

Kale/collard greens

Make the effort to buy organic food as often as you can. Not only is it good for you and your family, but it's also good for the planet.

REAL TIME CHANGE

I am beyond thrilled that I signed up for this program. It has been life changing for me. I never thought I could feel this great. It was truly effective. I never in a million years would have thought "eating clean" could feel this good.

I went into this thinking, "How can I give up sugar, carbs, and caffeine?" The healthy clean options were above my expectations, and I was completely satisfied. It has truly been a gift.

MARY LAMPE SUDDELL
NORTHPORT, NEW YORK

ME: Love your enthusiasm! Four years after my first cleanse, I remain as excited as ever about it. It's hard to believe that doing so little can make you feel so good.

A FISHY STORY

You couldn't eat fish during the cleanse, because sadly many types of fish have been contaminated by mercury, one of the most poisonous natural substances on the planet. That was a hardship for me, because I love sushi. Fish and shellfish contain high-quality protein and other essential nutrients, are low in saturated fat, and contain omega-3 fatty acids, but the bad news is that nearly all fish and shellfish contain traces of mercury. Factories that use coal for fuel pollute the atmosphere with mercury, which eventually finds its way into lakes, rivers, and the ocean, where it gets into the marine food chain. The fish absorb the mercury when they feed on organisms living in the water. The mercury binds to tissue in the fish, which is passed all the way up the food chain as big fish eat smaller ones. Mercury accumulates in the larger predator fish, which is why large fish are generally riskier to eat than smaller ones.

Eating too much fish contaminated by mercury can cause reproductive troubles, nervous system disorders, and liver impairment. I was horrified when I read that the Natural Resources Defense Council reports one in 13 American women of childbearing age carry enough mercury in their bloodstreams to put their unborn children at increased risk for developmental problems. This is a serious threat to the health of future generations.

Mercury binds to the tissues, especially in the kidneys and liver, and builds up over time. It damages the liver and leads to nonalcoholic fatty liver disease. To stay healthy, you want your liver to be in tip-top shape. You have to protect your liver. **You can eat low-mercury fish on the Clean Up Your Act Diet, but limit yourself to two portions of no more than 6 ounces a week.** The Natural Resources Defense Council has compiled a list of fish and shellfish and their mercury levels, which I include below. If you have the information, you can make the healthiest choices when you eat fish and seafood.

Lowest Mercury Levels

Enjoy these fish up to twice a week.

Anchovies	Mullet
Butterfish	Oyster
Catfish	Perch (ocean)
Clam	Plaice
Crab (domestic)	Pollock
Crawfish/Crayfish	Salmon (canned)**
Croaker (Atlantic)	Salmon (fresh)**
Flounder*	Sardine
Haddock (Atlantic)*	Scallop*
Hake	Shad (American)
Herring	Shrimp*
Mackerel (North Atlantic, chub)	Sole (Pacific)

Squid (calamari)

Tilapia

Trout (freshwater)

Whitefish

Whiting

Moderate Mercury Levels

Eat no more than four servings per month of these.

Bass (striped, black)

Carp

Cod (Alaskan)*

Croaker (White Pacific)

Halibut (Atlantic)*

Halibut (Pacific)

Jacksmelt (silverside)

Lobster

Mahi mahi

Monkfish*

Perch (freshwater)

Sablefish

Skate*

Snapper*

Tuna (canned chunk light)

Tuna (skipjack)*

Weakfish (sea trout)

High Mercury

Eat no more than two servings a month of these.

Bluefish

Grouper*

Mackerel (Spanish, gulf)

Sea Bass (Chilean)*

Tuna (canned albacore)

Tuna (yellowfin)*

Highest Mercury

Avoid eating these altogether.

Mackerel (king)

Marlin*

Orange roughy*

Shark*

Swordfish*

Tilefish*

Tuna (bigeye, ahi)*

* **Fish in trouble!** *The fish with an asterisk by their names are perilously low in numbers or are caught using environmentally destructive methods.*

** **Farmed salmon** *may contain PCBs, chemicals with serious long-term health effects.*

CLEAN UP YOUR ACT MEALS

When I am feeding myself, I don't want to spend a lot of time in the kitchen. I like to make things with leftovers I use for another meal. I sometimes double recipes and freeze what's left. Having a freezer stocked with veggie burgers, gluten-free pizza dough, quinoa, and soups makes it easy to put together a meal quickly. Though I'll give you 2 weeks of plans for the Clean Up Your Act Diet, I think it's important for you to own this way of eating. To keep on track, you have to find food that satisfies your taste. To be honest, I have my tried-and-true foods. I do better without a lot of variety. I don't mind eating the same things for days on end—especially when I'm busy. Almond butter on rice cakes; quinoa mixed with olive oil, garlic, and capers; a "kitchen sink" salad made with what's in the refrigerator; grilled chicken paillard or steak with a green salad; and berries all make me happy. When I'm pressed for time, I pick up an organic rotisserie chicken at the market and use the meat in different ways for a couple of days.

I've put together an overview of how to eat on the plan, with suggestions for breakfast, lunch, dinner, snacks, and desserts. **Reminder:** Keep your daily calorie consumption to 1,300 calories if you want to lose weight.

Breakfast Ideas

- Gluten-free oatmeal with cinnamon or fruit
- Cream of rice or cream of quinoa with rice or almond milk, berries, bananas, apple slices, and cinnamon
- Quinoa with blueberries and a drop of maple syrup
- Hard-boiled eggs
- Poached eggs on a bed of spinach, quinoa, or chili
- Coddled or baked eggs
- Omelets or scrambles with spinach and goat cheese, any combination of tomatoes, mushrooms, peppers, onions, broccoli, leeks, shallots, scallions, asparagus, black beans, smoked salmon, arugula, or fresh herbs—I especially like chives, cilantro, dill, and oregano. I throw whatever I have left over from the previous night into my omelets or on my eggs.
- Toppings for eggs and omelets: guacamole, tomato or mango salsa, leftover chili

- Gluten-free, low-sugar granola with rice milk or on goat or sheep yogurt
- Breakfast wrap made with gluten-free wraps, fried or scrambled eggs, assorted vegetables, beans, avocado, hot sauce, a slice of turkey
- Cantaloupe and other melons, berries, pineapple, or any fruit but citrus
- Fruit salad and sheep or goat yogurt
- Continue with a protein shake with fruit—starting your day with protein will keep you feeling full longer.

REAL TIME CHANGE

In the beginning, I was hating the shakes, but after the cleanse part, my husband and I decided we would still try to start the day or end it with smoothies instead of a meal.

AMY MURPHY
NEW YORK, NEW YORK

ME: Many people who do the cleanse want to continue with the protein shake for breakfast. It's a perfect breakfast—quick, nutritious, and sets you up for the day. People who start with a protein-rich breakfast win the hunger games later in the day.

Lunch or Dinner Ideas

- Wraps made with romaine or Boston lettuce, sliced turkey breast or roast beef, gluten-free wrap, or Asian rice wraps instead of bread: fill with hummus, carrots, celery, slices of avocado, asparagus, goat cheese, chicken, turkey, sliced beef, chopped nuts, cucumbers, salsa, beans
- Burgers: A burger doesn't have to be made of beef. You can use chopped chicken, turkey, lamb, salmon, tuna, or mahi mahi. And, of course, there are great-tasting veggie burgers. You can smother your burger in caramelized onions, mushrooms, guacamole, tomato, lettuce, peppers, jalapeños, sprouts, red onion, pesto, watercress, sun-dried tomatoes, grilled eggplant and tomato sauce, hummus with feta and olive tapenade, herbed goat cheese with roasted red peppers and horseradish, or cucumber with fresh spinach leaves and salsa. It makes me hungry just thinking of all you can do with a burger.

- Salads: Be creative! Use the deeper greens and skip the iceberg—go for all sorts of lettuce, baby kale, spinach as a base and pile on vegetables such as peppers, snap peas, mushrooms, artichoke hearts, olives, beans, tomatoes, shaved carrots, scallions, cauliflower, and zucchini. Add chicken, fish, scallops, shrimp, hard-boiled eggs, and nuts, pomegranate seeds, and chia seeds for crunch. Have fun building the salad and making dressings, too. As far as I'm concerned, there is nothing better than extra virgin olive oil and a squeeze of lemon or splash of vinegar (balsamic, cider, champagne, wine)—nothing that will overpower the flavor of the ingredients.

- Soup: Try not to eat soup from a can (unless it is organic and low salt). During the summer, making gazpacho from the tomatoes in my garden is a treat. I use organic, ready-made, low-sodium broths as a base if I'm in a hurry.

- One of my favorite soups is to add a can of organic white beans and some escarole to chicken or vegetable stock. It's an effortlessly nutritious soup.

- I make Italian *stracciatella* soup by adding chopped organic spinach and egg whites—or a whole lightly beaten egg—to low-sodium, organic chicken broth.

- I sometimes mash white beans and add chopped tomatoes, then splash a little balsamic vinegar on the mix.

- If you have run out of frozen soups, you can always find fresh soups to go at take-out restaurants and food stores before you make another batch. Try to find places that use organic vegetables. Stay away from soups with a cream base or with noodles and pasta.

- Leftovers: If you cook extra for dinner the night before, you can enjoy leftovers for lunch. Chili can be reheated or used in a wrap; extra steamed veggies can be added to an omelet; slices of cold chicken can be eaten with salsa on top of a rice cake. If I make a quinoa dish for dinner, I eat it cold the next day for lunch.

- Sometimes I put roasted root veggies on gluten-free toast and top it off with a soft-boiled egg.

- A cold pasta salad—using gluten-free pasta—is always delicious. I use pesto or *chimichurri* sauce, or olive oil and fresh herbs, and toss with raw or cooked vegetables.

Dinner Ideas

My rule of thumb is to have a protein and veggies for dinner. I keep it as simple as possible. Of course, it all depends on how hungry you are. If I have a big lunch, then a light dinner is all I need.

- My grill pan saves the day. I grill chicken, fish, steak, chicken sausage, or lamb chops on top of the stove and make sides of steamed, roasted, or grilled vegetables.
- Roasting a chicken or turkey breast will give you several meals.
- Loretta Lang Stokes came up with a chicken tenders recipe that will satisfy a craving and make your family happy. Just brush thinly cut pieces of chicken breast with a little olive oil and coat with almond meal. "Fry" the tenders in the oven on a parchment-covered baking sheet at 350°F. Turn the pieces after 10 minutes and brown the other side.
- Half a baked sweet potato is always a treat. I also make oven-baked sweet potato "fries," which I roast as I would any veggie. A sprinkle of maple syrup makes them even more delicious.
- A stir-fry is a quick meal—vegetables, thinly sliced chicken or beef, shrimp, or scallops with fresh ginger or hot sauce make a tasty meal. I use roasted sesame oil, rice vinegar, and sesame seeds for Asian flavor.
- You can make quinoa as a side dish or main course. I know I've said it before, but I love quinoa with olive oil, garlic, and capers—you've got to try it. It's a simple dish that works for me. There are several recipes that use quinoa in the No-Fuss Recipes.
- Now that you can eat gluten-free pasta, you can be creative with simple sauces or olive oil, vegetables, herbs, and nuts. Pasta with a salad is a very satisfying dinner, but no more than twice a week.
- Grill or roast a veggie mix of cauliflower, beans, broccoli—you name it— as a side or a main course.
- I make beef, turkey, or vegetable chili and freeze some to eat another day.
- I love meat loaf and meatballs. I use gluten-free oats or gluten-free bread crumbs to bind the meat.

Snacks

My snacks are usually mini-meals. The time of day doesn't dictate what I eat. I've been known to go through an entire container of blueberries in one sitting. Here is what I like to snack on:

- Olives
- Raw vegetables with hummus or guacamole
- Almond butter on rice cakes, celery, or slices of banana
- Nuts and seeds, including almonds, cashews, pecans, walnuts, and pumpkin seeds
- Marinated artichoke hearts
- Crispy roasted vegetables
- Kale chips
- Hard-boiled eggs—sometimes I scoop out the yoke, fill it with hummus, and sprinkle with paprika for really healthy deviled eggs
- Leftover quinoa, sweet or savory
- A slice of turkey, roast beef, or roast chicken
- Roll-ups—a lettuce leaf or a slice of turkey or roast beef filled with hummus, vegetables, or whatever I have around
- Fruits of all sorts—bananas, apples, pears, berries, melon, or pineapple (which is great grilled)
- A cup of soup
- Gluten-free crackers with goat cheese
- Mushroom Pâté (page 187) on a gluten-free cracker, in a wrap, or as a veggie dip
- Eggplant dip used the same way as the mushroom pate
- Chia seed bars

Desserts

If I crave something sweet, I go for fruit. Dessert can be a challenge, especially if you are a baker. Gluten-free baking is a category in itself. There are many gluten-free baking cookbooks on the shelves that you might want to look at. But cake is cake and cookies are cookies. You want to break out of that addiction. You'll find some delicious dessert recipes in Chapter 10, No-Fuss Recipes.

- Watermelon with feta, mint, and aged balsamic vinegar (I love this and eat it all the time!)
- Chia seed pudding (see recipes on pages 220 and 221)
- Ice Pops (see recipes starting on page 226) made with fresh fruit
- Grilled peaches, plums, pineapple
- A small portion of 70 percent chocolate

REAL TIME CHANGE

I am more conscious about what I put in my mouth. I want to take full advantage of where this cleanse has brought me. I read labels, cook as organic as I can, and stay away from gluten, dairy, sugar, alcohol, and caffeine. I have always been a good planner, so I have embraced planning my meals and have learned to adapt when going out to eat.

LORETTA LANG STOKES
BEVERLY, MASSACHUSETTS

ME: That's the spirit! It just takes a little planning to lock in the good habits you've formed.

STAY CLEAN WITH CLEANSING FOOD

You don't have to be on a cleanse to incorporate foods in your daily menu that will detox your body and cleanse your liver. These foods will give your liver a helping hand so that it works at peak efficiency all the time to keep you clean from the inside out.

30 Cleansing Foods That Will Keep Your Body Clean

1. Apples: the fiber pectin helps detox metals and food additives
2. Artichokes: increase bile production
3. Asparagus: a natural diuretic that helps with liver drainage

4. Avocados: contain glutathione, which helps the liver detoxify synthetic chemicals

5. Basil: helps the metabolic breakdown and elimination of chemicals in the blood

6. Beets: contain a mix of phytochemicals and minerals that make them great blood purifiers and liver cleansers

7. Brazil nuts: packed with selenium, which is vital in flushing mercury from your body

8. Broccoli: increases glutathione, which helps the liver transform toxins into a form that can be easily eliminated

9. Brussels sprouts: high in sulfur, which helps to remove toxins from the blood

10. Cabbage: also contains sulfur and stimulates the activation of two crucial liver detoxifying enzymes

11. Carrots: rich in glutathione

12. Cauliflower: aids production of enzymes that flush out toxins and carcinogens

13. Cilantro (coriander): helps mobilize mercury and other heavy metals out of the tissue so that the metals can attach to other compounds and be excreted from the body

14. Collard greens: have high cleansing properties

15. Dandelions: act on the liver by straining and filtering toxins and waste from the bloodstream; dandelion root tea has been shown to rid the liver of toxins

16. Fennel: protects the liver from harmful chemicals

17. Flaxseeds: when ground, provide fiber that helps to bind and flush out toxins from the intestinal tract; flax fiber suppresses appetite and helps support weight loss

18. Garlic: is loaded with sulfur

19. Ginger: spikes your metabolism, helps to flush out waste, and supports liver functions

20. Kale: provides comprehensive support for the entire detoxification system

21. Lemons: help to convert toxins into a water-soluble form that can be easily excreted from the body

22. Cold-pressed organic oils: including olive, hemp, and flaxseed, which provide a lipid base that can suck up harmful toxins

23. Onions: packed with sulfur-containing amino acids that detox the liver, taking some of the burden off that hardworking organ

24. Parsley: a diuretic herb that keeps your plumbing system running smoothly, helping to excrete toxins

25. Pineapples: contain bromelain, a digestive enzyme that helps to cleanse your colon

26. Spinach: raw spinach has a heavy dose of glutathione

27. Turmeric: the active ingredient is curcumin, which is used to treat liver and digestive disorders in Ayurvedic medicine

28. Walnuts: hold high levels of acid arginine, which aids the liver in detoxifying ammonia, as well as glutathione

29. Watercress: has a cleansing action that helps to release enzymes in the liver that get rid of toxic buildup

30. Wheatgrass: restores alkalinity to the blood and is a powerful detoxer and liver protector

---

REAL TIME CHANGE

I think that if I can continue to honor how my body feels and not stuff my face with something gross because it satisfies my tastebuds, I will be able to stick to it. It's a funny distinction—momentary satisfaction vs. long-term, whole body feeling—and one that I need to value/hear/honor.

MICHELE BLOOM
SOUTH ORANGE, NEW JERSEY

ME: You put this so well—momentary satisfaction vs. long-term, whole body feeling. To be honest, I choose momentary satisfaction every once in a while, but not often enough to wreck the hard work I've done to be in good shape in body, mind, and spirit.

Do your best to eat some of these foods each day. If you do, you are giving your body a daily cleaning service. You've worked hard to reduce your toxic load. Now it's your job to stay clean. It's easy if you do a little every day to tidy up. You need to support your body in doing what it does naturally.

Okay! You know what you have to do. Remember, it took you a long time to get where you are. Be patient. Slow and steady—change will happen. You will achieve the goals you set or find new, even better ones.

You have the basics now, but when it comes to being out there in the world, some practical advice will smooth the way for you. The next chapter will give you tips on how to make the Clean Up Your Act Diet work anywhere—when you travel, eat out at restaurants or at the homes of friends and family. You'll need strategies to get through cocktail parties, other social events, and the holidays without going crazy with the wrong foods. We even give you a one-day mini-cleanse just in case you lose it now and then.

Age is an issue of mind over matter. If you don't mind, it doesn't matter.
—MARK TWAIN

9

Any Time, Any Place: Practical Tips to Make It Work

On a 2-week whirlwind in New York that included meeting at Rodale's office with the terrific women who had signed on to try the cleanse, I also fractured two fingers while doing extreme gardening, did the photo shoot for the book cover without the cast on my fingers—ouch!—celebrated my daughter Stella's college graduation, and spent time with my delicious granddaughter. I'm always pleasantly surprised by how easy it's become for me to stay on track food-wise, even with all the craziness. It's just automatic now, and I love that. These days, the taste of junk food disgusts me, and nutrition-dense, fresh food is what I crave. I know if you stick with this, it will be the same for you! So keep up the good work. Being mindful about what you eat will pay off.

Supermarket Finds

I prowl the aisles at Whole Foods and Trader Joe's on the lookout for products that work on the Clean Up Your Act Diet. I have to say the choices have grown a lot in just the 4 years I've been eating this way. I was in a Stop & Shop recently and was surprised at the selection of gluten-free products they had. What was great is they had everything I needed in one or two aisles. I didn't have to hunt all over the store. Check your local supermarket. There is more there than you might think. These are some of the prepared foods you'll find in my kitchen cabinets:

Justin's Almond Butter: I love the little individual packets. I can slip a couple in my purse and have an easy snack on hand. When I get ravenous with no food in sight, I just tear open a packet and squeeze the almond butter into my mouth. Very elegant, right?

Mary's Gone Crackers: These gluten-free crackers come in a number of flavors, including original, herb, black pepper, super seed, onion, jalapeño, and caraway. Mary's also makes bread crumbs and pretzels.

Udi's has a full line of gluten-free baked goods, including tortillas, breads, rolls, pizza crust, and muffins. Your goal is to eat clean, so you should consider these products occasional treats. Udi's also makes great cookies, but remember—just because they're gluten-free does not mean they are low in calories. You should approach these as you would any cookie. Along with the standard oatmeal raisin, chocolate chip, and snickerdoodle cookies, Udi's makes maple pecan chocolate chip, peanut butter coconut, ginger, dark chocolate, and salted caramel cashew cookies.

Wow cookies: These are delicious but high in sugar. They come in chocolate chip, peanut butter, ginger molasses, snickerdoodle, and lemon burst. Be very careful about portion control.

Schar has a full line of gluten-free products, including pastas, crackers, and cookies. They make a variety of breads such as baguettes and ciabatta.

Ancient Harvest makes terrific gluten-free pastas and ancient grains blends. This is my go-to pasta brand.

Hodgson Mill has an entire line of gluten-free products, including flours, a seasoned coating mix, and pastas. There is a good selection of gluten-free mixes and milled flaxseed.

Bob's Red Mill has an impressive range of gluten-free flours and many other products for baking. This brand is a good source for gluten-free oats.

Food for Life makes brown rice and black rice tortillas that are great wraps. They also have brown rice English muffins that are gluten free. Check out their products.

Healthy Warrior makes delicious chia bars that are full of omega-3s and low in sugar in a variety of flavors: coconut, acai berry, chocolate peanut butter, banana nut, apple cinnamon, coffee, dark chocolate cherry, and mango. A perfect snack—and only 100 calories.

Mt. Sterling Co-op Creamery produces very good goat milk cheeses. They include a mild, sharp, and smoked Cheddar-style cheese; a mozzarella, which is great for pizza; and country jack cheese in a variety of flavors, including chives, dill, jalapeño, and olive and balsamic vinegar.

Woolwich Dairy Inc. is another great source of goat cheese, including mozzarella, brie, and Tre Fratello. The flavored chevres are sophisticated and delicious—for example, cranberry cinnamon, wild blueberry vanilla, fig, and bruschetta.

Granulated stevia should be in your new pantry. It's an herbal sugar substitute that you can use in the same measure as sugar, so you don't have to pull out a calculator to see how much you need to use. There are a number of brands available. Some of the best include: Stevia in the Raw, Stevita Spoonable Sweetener, NuNaturals NuStevia White Stevia Powder. See page 218 for a chart converting sugar to stevia.

Thomas Keller, the chef at French Laundry, one of the best restaurants in the country, has a line of products sold at Williams-Sonoma, including Ad Hoc Gluten-free Pancake and Waffle Mix, Cup 4 Cup Gluten-free Flour, Cup 4 Cup Gluten-free Brownie Mix, and Cup 4 Cup Gluten-free Pizza Crust Mix.

Earth Balance makes a soy-free vegan butter substitute as well as an organic coconut spread.

Vegenaise has two acceptable mayonnaise substitutes, Soy-Free Vegenaise and Grapeseed Oil Vegenaise, but use them sparingly.

When you see that there are many foods on the shelves that are on the plan, you won't feel so restricted. Just as you wouldn't indulge in your favorite cookies, don't go wild with gluten-free alternatives. You should still try to keep your diet to predominantly fresh, simple foods that are not packaged.

REAL TIME CHANGE

I miss sweets but am learning to live without them or limiting them. I will not put just anything in my mouth. A small square of dark chocolate will do the trick, whereas before the cleanse it might have been a sleeve of Oreos or box of Girl Scout cookies!

LORETTA LANG STOKES
BEVERLY, MASSACHUSETTS

ME: I love that you're making this plan your own. Once you've got the fundamentals down, you have to find your way to tailor the plan for you.

This chapter prepares you to be strong out there in the world. Whether you are at a supermarket or traveling, eating out or baking a cake, you need some guidance to apply the principles of the Clean Up Your Act Diet. Taking the guesswork out of making the right choices and positioning yourself to resist temptation will go a long way to making clean eating stress free.

14 DAYS OF CLEAN UP YOUR ACT DIET MEAL PLANS

We're including 2 weeks of meal plans to show you how easy and delicious eating clean can be. I haven't added beverages. You know to stay well-hydrated. You can add a cup of coffee a day if you'd like, but if you've done well without it, why start it up again? Dessert appears every fourth day, because I want you to consider dessert a treat, not a daily habit. If you have a sweet tooth and can keep your caloric consumption to 1,300, then go for it—as long as your desserts are gluten free, sugar free, and dairy free. In Chapter 10, you'll find a number of desserts you might want to try.

DAY 1

Breakfast: Quinoa with blueberries and a splash of maple syrup
Snack: Almond butter on rice cake
Lunch: Mediterranean Lettuce Wrap (page 199)
Snack: A cup of chicken soup from the freezer

Dinner: Grilled salmon with steamed asparagus with a hard-boiled egg crumbled on top (make extra asparagus and hard-boiled eggs)
Dessert: Vanilla or Chocolate Chia Seed Pudding (page 220 or 221)

DAY 2

Breakfast: Asparagus omelet with fresh dill
Snack: Pineapple
Lunch: Black Bean Soup (page 190; freeze some for the future)
Snack: Raw veggies and Hummus (see recipes starting on page 185)
Dinner: Veggie Burger (see recipes starting on page 201; freeze some for the future) with slices of avocado and tomato, lettuce, and Quinoa Tabbouleh (page 216)

DAY 3

Breakfast: Gluten-free oatmeal with berries
Snack: Healthy deviled eggs (see page 143)
Lunch: Sliced turkey wrap with a spoon of leftover Black Bean Soup, chopped tomato, and avocado
Snack: Chia seed bar
Dinner: My Slow Cooker Beef Stew (page 192; freeze some for the future) with green salad

DAY 4

Breakfast: Breakfast wrap with scrambled eggs, sweet peppers, and salsa
Snack: Fruit salad with sheep or goat yogurt
Lunch: Quinoa with olive oil, capers, and lemon
Snack: Mushroom Pâté (page 187) with raw vegetables, rice cakes, or gluten-free crackers
Dinner: Almond meal chicken tenders (see page 142) with a medley of sliced Roasted Veggies (page 212; make extra) such as red onion, Brussels sprouts, and squash and sweet potato oven fries
Dessert: Ice Pop (see recipes starting on page 226)

DAY 5

Breakfast: Gluten-free toast topped with leftover Roasted Veggies and a poached or soft-boiled egg

Snack: Plums or nectarines with a sprinkle of balsamic vinegar

Lunch: Leftover My Slow Cooker Beef Stew

Snack: Almond butter on apple slices

Dinner: Pizza (see recipes starting on page 206) and green salad

DAY 6

Breakfast: Protein shake with berries

Snack: Almond butter on celery

Lunch: Hamburger with lettuce, tomato, onion, and avocado and leftover Quinoa Tabbouleh

Snack: Gluten-free crackers with goat cheese

Dinner: Multitasking Vegetable Soup (page 191; freeze some for the future)

DAY 7

Breakfast: Omelet with a big spoonful of veggies from Multitasking Vegetable Soup

Snack: Watermelon, feta, and mint

Lunch: Layered roast beef wrap with hummus, leftover Mushroom Pate, carrots, celery, and pepper sticks

Snack: Mixed nuts

Dinner: Roasted chicken (see recipes on pages 193 and 194; save some white meat for lunch) with spaghetti squash (save some undressed "spaghetti" for future) with pesto

Dessert: Pear and Ginger Crumble (page 225)

DAY 8

Breakfast: Protein shake with banana

Snack: Hard-boiled egg

Lunch: Waldorf salad with leftover chicken, apples, walnuts, celery, and lettuce

Snack: Kale chips

Dinner: Lamb chops with a green bean and quinoa salad

DAY 9

Breakfast: Gluten-free granola with rice or almond milk

Snack: Leftover spaghetti squash with olive oil and garlic

Lunch: Stracciatella soup (page 141) with a green salad with artichoke hearts

Snack: White Bean Puree (page 188) with veggies

Dinner: Poached or grilled chicken breasts (make one for tomorrow's lunch), ½ baked sweet potato, and steamed broccoli

DAY 10

Breakfast: Oatmeal with cinnamon and walnuts

Snack: Cup of stracciatella soup

Lunch: Sliced chicken breast added to a green bean and quinoa salad

Snack: Mixed berries

Dinner: Winter Squash and Bean Stew (page 196)

DAY 11

Breakfast: Diced honeydew, sliced almonds with lime juice

Snack: Winter Squash and Bean Stew

Lunch: Greek salad with diced tomatoes, cucumbers, red onion, and feta with oregano

Snack: Hummus with raw veggies

Dinner: Shrimp boil (use Old Bay Seasoning; save some for a snack) with mashed white beans, chopped tomatoes, and a splash of balsamic vinegar

Dessert: Biscotti (pages 218 and 219)

DAY 12

Breakfast: Fruit salad sprinkled with gluten-free granola

Snack: Almond butter on a rice cake

Lunch: Diced hard-boiled eggs mixed with diced avocado, salsa, and fresh cilantro

Snack: Shrimp cocktail with white horseradish

Dinner: Stir-fry with sliced beef, sweet peppers, onions, snow peas, mushrooms, carrot sticks, sesame seeds, and a splash of sesame oil

Breakfast: Protein shake with peaches

Snack: Marinated artichoke hearts

Lunch: Simple Chicken Soup (page 189)

Snack: White Bean Puree (page 188) and raw veggies

Dinner: Chicken paillard with arugula salad on top

Breakfast: Vegetable Frittata with Quinoa (page 198)

Snack: Pear

Lunch: Turkey or veggie burger with black beans and guacamole

Snack: Olives

Dinner: Quinoa pasta tossed with thinly sliced red pepper, broccoli florets, and pesto

Dessert: Ice Pop (see recipes starting on page 226)

READ THE SMALL PRINT

Not all food in boxes, cans, and bags is bad for you. Food manufacturers have responded to the growing demand for healthy food by producing some very good products. Last year, Lisa, Monica, and I went to a healthy food exhibition at the giant convention center in Anaheim. It was unbelievable! There were rows and rows of booths in several rooms, each one pitching a product or a line of products. Confession: I did try way too many samples and went home carrying bags of them. Some things tasted like cardboard—really awful! But there were many products I would enjoy again.

You know not to be tricked by the promises and buzzwords, which are so often marketing ploys to seduce you into buying the product. "Lite" or "light" might be misleading. "Low fat" or "fat free" does not mean that the sugar content isn't too high. "No added sugar"—as in sucrose—might be true, but the product might still have natural sugars. The only way to know if a processed food is the right choice is to study the nutrition label carefully, which can be a pain if you have to wear reading glasses but is absolutely worth it. I wouldn't buy anything from the center aisles of the supermarket without checking out the nutritional information and the ingredients.

Start with the serving size, the number of calories in a single serving, and the number of servings in the package. Before I became a more conscious eater, I could eat several servings of most things without blinking an eye. You have to decide if you can limit your portion size and if the calorie count is worth it. Many times I put a package back on the shelf because the food is no caloric bargain.

Moving down the label, I look at the fat content. The "Total Fat" refers to saturated, polyunsaturated, monounsaturated, and trans fats. Foods that call themselves "trans fat free" can contain up to a half gram of trans fats per serving. Look out for hydrogenated oils and partially hydrogenated oils, which are the primary sources of trans fats.

Saturated fat and trans fats have to be broken out.

- Products with 20 g per 100 g of fat or less are acceptable.
- Saturated fats should be less than 5 g per 100 g.
- Put back any product that contains trans fats.

Nutrition Facts		
Serving Size		
Servings Per Container		
Amount Per Serving		
Calories 0	Calories from Fat 0	
		% Daily Value*
Total Fat 0g		0%
Saturated Fat 0g		0%
Trans Fat 0g		
Cholesterol 0mg		0%
Sodium 0mg		0%
Total Carbohydrate 0g		0%
Dietary Fiber 0g		0%
Soluble Fiber 0g		0%
Insoluble Fiber 0g		0%
Sugars 0g		
Protein 0g		
Vitamin A 0%	•	Vitamin C 0%
Calcium 0%	•	Iron 0%
Phosphorus 0%	•	Magnesium 0%

* Percent Daily Values are based on a 2,000 calorie diet. Your daily values may be higher or lower depending on your calorie needs:

		Calories:	2,000	2,500
Total Fat	Less than		0g	0g
Sat Fat	Less than		0g	0g
Cholesterol	Less than		0mg	0mg
Sodium	Less than		0mg	0mg
Potassium			0mg	0mg
Total Carbohydrate			0g	0g
Dietary Fiber			0g	0g

Calories per gram:
Fat 0 • Carbohydrate 0 • Protein 0

INGREDIENTS: Whole Wheat Flour, (Stone Ground Whole Oats, Hard Red Winter Wheat, Rye, Long Grain Brown Rice, Triticale, Buckwheat, Barley, Sesame Seeds), Malted Barley, Salt, Yeast, Mixed Tocopherols (Natural Vitamin E) for Freshness.
CONTAINS WHEAT INGREDIENTS

DISTRIBUTED BY
COMPANY NAME
ADDRESS
CITY, STATE, ZIP
WEB ADDRESS

Next, look at the sodium line. Sodium has several names, including salt, sodium benzoate, disodium or monosodium glutamate (MSG), sodium nitrate, and sodium nitrite. More on the last two later. Sodium content should be under 600 mg. Low sodium is 140 mg or less. I go for low sodium, because I like to use my Celtic sea salt.

The next line covers carbohydrates: sugars, starches, and fibers. This is where you run into trouble on the Clean Up Your Act Diet. You will have to check the ingredient list carefully, because of the restrictions. **The thing to remember**

is that there are 4 to 5 calories for each gram of sugar, so you can calculate how many calories per serving derive from sugar.

- You should try to choose products with no more than 5 g of sugar. Since you are supposed to be off added sugar completely, even a sugar content that low is a treat.
- Whole grain foods should deliver at least 3 g of fiber per serving. Look for a high fiber content, which would be at least 5 g.

Your next concern is the ingredients, which are listed in descending order of quantity. The first two or three ingredients are the ones that matter most. Ingredients at the bottom of the list may appear in tiny amounts. Still, even tiny amounts of toxins accumulate in your body. That's why I try to avoid buying anything with an ingredient I can't pronounce.

The list of aliases for sugar on page 39 will tell you the many names that fructose, sucrose, and dextrose go by. Remember, do not buy a product with an ingredient ending in -ose in the top three. Forget about artificial sweeteners—these man-made chemicals trick your body and screw up your metabolism.

Beyond the gluten-free label, remember you are staying away from dairy and soy products.

If you are eating clean, all the chemicals that are extending the shelf life of the product or compensating for processing are not for you.

REAL TIME CHANGE

I read the labels more often. I think about what I'm about to consume more than I ever did before. I catch myself eating when I really don't need to, and stop myself.

ILIANA GUIBERT
NEW YORK, NEW YORK

ME: Soon finding foods that work for you will become second nature. It becomes easy to decide which packaged foods are just not good for you. Now that you're eating clean, that stuff won't taste good anymore. You can taste the chemicals. It just doesn't do it for me anymore.

Put It Back on the Shelf If You See These Ingredients

As you inspect the ingredient list on food labels, handle a package like a hot potato if any of these chemicals are listed:

Sodium nitrite and sodium nitrate are used as preservatives in meats. They may pose a cancer risk. Bye-bye, little franks in a blanket.

Food dyes or artificial colorings are added to processed food to suggest a relationship with the food in its original state or to appeal to children. The dyes hide the drab colors of heavily processed food. They appear on the ingredient list by their color name, such as Yellow 5 or Blue 1. The food industry makes caramel coloring by treating sugar with ammonia, which creates carcinogens. It's a good thing you've given up colas.

Hydrolyzed vegetable protein, a flavor enhancer, is a plant protein that has been broken down to amino acids. One of the amino acids, glutamate acid, joins with sodium in your body to form monosodium glutamate, better known as MSG, an additive that causes headaches, nausea, and other adverse reactions. MSG is listed as an ingredient when it is added to products directly, but when it is a by-product of hydrolyzed protein, it does not appear on the label.

BHA is used as a preservative to keep food that contains oil from going rancid. Though animal testing has shown that it causes cancer in studies, it has not been banned.

Parabens are synthetic preservatives that are used to stop the growth of mold and yeast in foods. They disrupt your hormonal balance and have been found in breast cancer tissue.

BPA (bisphenol A). This plastic hardener is used in plastic bottles, food can liners, and cash register receipts. BPA has been linked to increased heart disease, cancer, and sexual dysfunction. Some companies have begun to phase out BPA-lined cans.

These examples are only the tip of the iceberg. You have to be aware of, or beware, the chemical ingredients in packaged food, most of which have never been tested.

Substitutions

When you think about cooking, you may be baffled about what you can do to replace flour, bread crumbs, butter, milk, and sugar. Remember, you will still be avoiding soy products, which limits some of the vegan substitutes on the market. There are a number of very good cookbooks available that will teach you some tricks and give you ideas. It's a whole new world, which is why I keep it simple and close to the source. If you are more ambitious than I am, here are some ideas for replacements you can use on the plan.

Flours

A blend of several flours is needed to get the same texture as wheat flour. There are dozens of flours that are gluten free. Light, starchy gluten-free flours include sweet rice flour, white rice flour, and starches such as tapioca starch, potato starch, and arrowroot starch. For medium flours, which are like all-purpose flours, the best tasting is sorghum, also called sweet sorghum or jowar flour. Gluten-free oat flour is also very good. Brown rice flour is better for baking than plain rice flour, which has a gummy feel in the mouth. The heavier grains have more protein: quinoa, millet, buckwheat nut meal, and bean/legume flours. These flours are like baking with whole wheat flour. Chickpea flour can boost protein and lower carbs, but it is best mixed with other flours. Coconut flour is rich in fiber and highly absorbent, so you will need to use more oil or liquid in a recipe. Almond meal or flour is a rich substitute that adds protein and omega-3s to baked goods.

I'm including the three recipes for gluten-free flours just in case some of you like to bake. Baking without gluten, sugar, and dairy takes ingenuity, but it can be done. We do include several baking recipes in Chapter 10. The fact is that there are some gluten-free flours on the market now that will do the trick, but they can be expensive. You might want to mix your own. I found these flour blends in *Simply Gluten Free Magazine*, which you should take a look at. They have great recipes and advice.

In the following flour blend recipes, you may not be familiar with one of the ingredients—xanthan gum. Xanthan gum is a plant-based thickening and stabilizing agent. For the record, it is a form of sugar. Xanthan gum works as an emulsifier that allows unfriendly liquids to mix. It helps to thicken liquids and batters and can create a creamy texture.

ALL-PURPOSE GLUTEN-FREE FLOUR BLEND

Use as you would all-purpose wheat flour. If yeast is an ingredient in the recipe, add ¾ teaspoon xanthan gum per cup of flour called for in the recipe.

4½ cups white rice flour

1½ cups sweet rice flour

2 cups potato starch (not potato flour)

1 cup tapioca starch

4 teaspoons xanthan gum

Whisk all the ingredients together well. Store in an airtight container.

HIGH-PROTEIN GLUTEN-FREE FLOUR BLEND

This works well for pie crust, bread, and other baked goods. For recipes with yeast, add ½ teaspoon xanthan gum per cup of flour called for in the recipe.

2¼ cups chickpea flour

2 cups superfine brown rice flour

2 cups potato starch

2 cups tapioca starch

4 teaspoons xanthan gum

Whisk all the ingredients together well. Store in an airtight container.

HIGH-FIBER GLUTEN-FREE FLOUR BLEND

This is a nutritious flour blend with extra fiber. When yeast is a recipe ingredient, add ½ teaspoon xanthan gum per cup of flour called for in the recipe.

2 cups superfine brown rice flour

2 cups sweet white sorghum flour

1⅓ cups tapioca starch

⅔ cup potato starch

3 teaspoons xanthan gum

Whisk all the ingredients together well. Store in an airtight container.

Other Substitutes

Milk: Unsweetened rice milk, almond milk, coconut milk. To replace full-fat milk, add one egg yolk for each cup of milk you need in rice milk or filtered water.

Buttermilk: Add 1 tablespoon lemon juice or 1 tablespoon apple cider vinegar to 1 cup rice or hemp milk. Allow the mixture to sour for 5 minutes.

Heavy cream: Mix ⅔ cup dairy-free milk of choice and ⅓ cup melted vegan butter or coconut oil.

Yogurt: 1 cup fruit puree or 1 cup unsweetened applesauce

Butter (one stick): ⅓ cup of any of the following: raw coconut oil, extra virgin olive oil (not for baking), unsweetened applesauce, pureed avocado, or mashed bananas. There are also a number of vegan spreads that are gluten and soy free.

Gluten-free bread crumbs: Gluten-free oats, day-old gluten-free bread, flax-seeds, or almonds zapped in a food processor or blender. There are several gluten-free bread crumbs on the market now, but be sure to check the label.

Soy sauce substitute: Bragg Liquid Aminos

You do not have to become a hermit chained to your kitchen for the rest of your life to follow the Clean Up Your Act Diet. I'll walk you through a variety of situations that might challenge your resolve. In time, you will develop your own routines for dealing with temptations at parties, during the holidays, at restaurants, eating your favorite cuisine, or while traveling for business or pleasure. There is a great big world of good food out there. You can be discriminating as easily as you can be out of control.

REAL TIME CHANGE

Transitioning to the everyday eating plan was not difficult, but if you were going out or to someone else's house to eat, it was challenging. My family would make something specifically for us, which was supportive.

AMY MURPHY
NEW YORK, NEW YORK

ME: You're lucky that your family is so good to you! Appreciate them every day, which I'm sure you do.

HOW TO SURVIVE COCKTAIL AND DINNER PARTIES
AND FESTIVE OCCASIONS

At home, you've got the logistics of eating clean down. You buy the right foods, cook your meals, and dole out reasonable portions. Social events and holidays can trip you up if you're not careful. Not only are you surrounded by high-calorie food and tons of sweets, but you also don't want to insult your host or succumb to peer pressure. There are a number of things you can do to keep up the good work despite the temptations.

Cocktail parties are extremely dangerous, and so is the premeal cocktail hour. Hors d'oeuvres look so small and innocuous, but those treats can be incredibly high in calories. I've been known to consume a day's worth of calories by eating all sorts of things wrapped in flaky pastry or full of crème fraiche. By the time I leave the party, I don't even feel full—I'm ready to go out to dinner! Just because you are not sitting down for a full meal at a cocktail party does not protect you from overindulging. Here are a few strategies I use to get through these events and remain mindful of what I eat:

- On arriving, I do a walk-through of the party and get an idea of what is being served at stations or passed on trays. I can plan what I want to eat. I use this time to say hello to friends, family, and business associates.
- I start with ice water and do not touch food for about 15 minutes. If I start eating and drinking right away, it's easy to overdo it.
- I place myself as far away from the hors d'oeuvres as I can. I circulate and focus on the people, not the food.
- If I'm going to drink, I avoid mixed drinks, which can be calorie bombs, and have a glass of wine instead.
- For every drink I have, I have a glass of water, which fills me up.

Dinner at the home of friends or family presents another level of temptations that can lure you away from your eating plan. I have some tricks up my sleeve for handling a dinner party without falling off the wagon.

- If I know my host, I find out the menu in advance so that I can plan my meal.
- Sometimes I offer to bring a healthy dish that I know I can eat.

- I don't arrive hungry. Instead I have a snack an hour or two before leaving home.

- During the evening, I don't talk about the way I eat now unless asked. My host has gone to a lot of trouble to prepare the meal. I do not want to take the guests' attention away from the food.

- When hors d'oeuvres and drinks are served, I stay away from the salty munchies and the gooey cheeses. I'm so happy to see a platter of crudités. I stick with water with lemon or lime and wait to have a glass of wine when we sit for dinner.

- If dinner is served family style or with passed platters, I help myself to the veggies, salads, and meats and just put a drop of rich sauces on the side. When dinner is served this way, you can pass on simple carbs. If dinner is plated, dig in to the healthy food, and just sample the food you want to avoid. Sometimes a friend's signature dish—like vegetable lasagna—is irresistible, but a few bites are enough to satisfy me.

- You can rearrange what's left on your plate so that it appears you have eaten more. I spend most of my energy talking and laughing with the other dinner guests. That's the point, isn't it?

- When it comes to dessert, I usually say, "The meal was absolutely delicious—I can't eat another bite," which is usually true. If I can't resist a fabulous treat, I exercise the four-bite rule. I make sure to eat those bites slowly and to savor every morsel! Otherwise, I go for the fruit, which is so often served these days.

- When people are indulging, they want you to join them and can be persistent if you try to pass on their favorite dessert. You can make it easy on yourself and turn the situation around by saying, "I'm stuffed, but that looks so great I can't resist having a bite." You're fine as long as you don't gobble it down.

It just takes having the right mind-set to make the evening fun instead of a battle between your willpower and your cravings.

'Tis the season to be jolly . . . I love celebrating Christmas and have a big party on Christmas Day known far and wide for the bingo we play. I collect prizes for an entire year—most of them "As Seen on TV" gadgets. I take my bingo seriously. We

REAL TIME CHANGE

I had a setback this past weekend. I was away for the weekend to attend a Sweet Sixteen birthday party in Florida for my best friend's daughter. I did very well on Thursday, Friday, and part of the day on Saturday, because as soon as I got there, I asked my friend to take me food shopping for the essentials to keep me on track.

The party was on Saturday night. The bad news is I drank alcohol and ate the food they served—chicken breast, potatoes, and yellow rice with vegetables. It was a small portion. The good news: I drank water in between the drinks, and I danced a lot. I ran out of the shake on Saturday morning. On Sunday morning, my best friend invited her whole family over for breakfast. I did not overeat, even though it was tempting. I got back on Sunday night after midnight and resumed the routine.

ANA NAPOLES
BLOOMFIELD, NEW JERSEY

ME: You couldn't have handled this situation better. You went off plan but were careful not to go too far by watching your portions, drinking a lot of water, and moving. Then you got right back on that horse! Congratulations!

have a blast! It's not just about the food, although there's plenty of good food. It's about the people, laughter, singing around the piano, a big fire in the fireplace. It's really lovely, a night filled with fun, warmth, and holiday spirit. Love it!

Holidays don't have to set off a feeding frenzy. One study showed that overweight people gain between 2.75 and 4 pounds during the 3 weeks around Christmas and often don't take it off. Another found that the average weight gain of adults from late September to early March is a pound. That may not seem like a lot, but most people don't lose that extra pound during the spring and summer, which means most people are going to gain 10 pounds each decade. That's one way our weight creeps up with age. This is what I do to make it through the holidays with my best intentions for healthy eating intact:

- I try to be consistent in my eating habits for most meals. I figure if I eat well 80 percent of the time and allow myself some treats 20 percent of the time, I'll be okay.

- I try to focus on my loved ones and doing fun things—like our now famous Christmas bingo—rather than the food.
- I often host parties so that I can control the menu and be certain there is plenty for me to eat.
- I make sure to exercise even more than usual. After a holiday meal, I go for a long walk with my family and my dog, Elsie.
- If the season feels stressful, I build in time alone to relax, even if it's only soaking in an Epsom salts bath.
- I prioritize what I want to splurge on. If I can't resist the stuffing, I bypass the cheese and crackers.
- I'm vigilant about portion sizes. If a number of dishes appeal to me, I take very small portions so that I get to taste everything.
- I eat slowly. It takes 20 minutes for our bodies to register that we are full. The more slowly I eat, the less food I'll eat. There is no reason to shovel down your food. Enjoy the company!
- I watch the drinking. Too much alcohol lowers my resistance.
- I'm careful about leftovers, which I store in small containers to avoid picking and overeating.
- If I'm having trouble staying on track, I keep a food log to be mindful of what I'm putting in my mouth.
- If I go astray, I get right back on track.

The holidays do not have to be a month of out-of-control eating and drinking. You will feel so much better if you maintain your commitment to healthy

REAL TIME CHANGE

I plan to do the cleanse at least twice a year. The first one I have planned will be in November, pre-holiday time as a way to keep on the right path during the holidays.

DIANE ARPINO
RAMSEY, NEW JERSEY

ME: That's good thinking. I like to do my annual cleanse in the summer, because there is so much delicious fresh food around.

eating. Celebrate with special activities rather than food. You can go skiing or ice-skating, attend a holiday concert, see some great movies, get a spa treatment, or all of the above. The holiday spirit involves a lot more than food! It is a time to enjoy the people you love and to be thankful for all the good in your life.

HOW TO STAY ON PLAN WHEN YOU'RE EATING OUT

We are eating away from home more and more. **Americans, on average, eat in a restaurant five times a week, according to a 2013 survey conducted by LivingSocial.** Aside from being too busy and tired to plan, cook, and clean up, we enjoy meeting friends or treating the family to a good meal out. But confronted by cocktails, the breadbasket, and a tempting menu, it's easy to throw all caution to the wind and eat too much of the wrong things. To eat healthy when you eat out, you have to be prepared. This game plan keeps my eating under control most of the time.

1. **Don't go out to eat famished.** I do eat smaller meals during the day if I'm having dinner out. But I make sure to have a small snack an hour before I leave the house, so I don't arrive ready to devour anything and everything.

2. **Check out the menu before you go.** Most restaurants post their menus on their Web sites, or you can go to MenuPages.com and similar Web sites to find out what the place is serving. Skip buffet restaurants—it's so hard not to overeat. Check out the dishes that look healthy, like grilled fish, poultry and meat, salads, and vegetable sides. It's a good idea to decide what you want to eat before you leave the house, and then you won't be tempted to try less healthy options. Watch out for menu buzzwords: "Battered" or "batter-dipped," "breaded," "with gravy," "cream sauce," "au gratin," and "smothered" are not for you. Stick to your decisions at the restaurant and don't be swayed by what others are ordering. If you decide you have to have that lasagna, then eat carefully during the day so at least your caloric intake does not go through the roof. Take a menu with you when you leave a restaurant so that you'll have a copy on hand when you return or order in.

3. **Make reservations.** This cuts down waiting and hunger-building time and the drinks you are tempted to have at the bar.

4. **Try to get a quiet table away from the kitchen.** If you are at a table with a lot of distractions, you will eat more, because you lose track of how much you're consuming. The bustle can make you eat more quickly. Sitting by the kitchen can be dangerous as you watch decadent dishes parade by. It's way too tempting.

5. **Don't have more than one drink.** Not only does drinking add calories, but it also does a number on your self-control. If you have a drink on an empty stomach, you are more likely to stray from the game plan. Drink water or a spicy Virgin Mary before your main course. You can order a drink or wine when some food arrives at the table. Of course, you have to splurge now and then—I have my two lychee martinis on Saturday night—but I am very careful about what I eat.

6. **Tell the cute guy with the breadbasket to walk on by.** All the free munchies that magically appear when you sit down—bread and rolls, popovers, tortilla chips, Chinese noodles, *pappadams*—are caloric disasters that lead to mindless eating when you are at your hungriest. Start drinking ice water right away.

7. **By special request.** You can have it your way at most restaurants. Don't hesitate to ask for items on the menu to be prepared as you would like. You can ask to drop some ingredients, such as cheese in a salad. You can ask if the chef will prepare the food with extra virgin olive oil. Sauces and dressings should always be served on the side. You can request that a dish be steamed, broiled, grilled, poached, or baked rather than fried. Substitute a steamed vegetable, salad, or baked potato for fries.

8. **Order appetizers or side dishes instead of a main course.** What's good about appetizers is that you don't have to worry about portion control. A starter and a salad can be a great meal. Broth-based soups, grilled vegetables, and seafood salads are the way to go. Beware cheesy, fried, creamy, and buttery choices.

9. **Don't fall into the salad trap.** All salads are not equal. Watch out for macaroni, potato, coleslaw, tuna, and chicken salads, which can be loaded with calories, mayonnaise, and sugar. Stick to fresh greens,

beans, and veggies and avoid the add-ons like bacon, cheese, croutons, and dried fruit that can turn a salad into a caloric disaster. Stick with vinaigrettes or fresh lemon for dressings. When the dressing is served on the side, measure out a small amount of dressing with your spoon. For a thicker dressing, dip your salad fork in the dressing and then help yourself to a bite of salad.

10. **Don't clean your plate.** Many restaurants serve huge portions of food. Just because it's in front of you doesn't mean you have to eat until you're stuffed. Stop when you feel satisfied. If a restaurant serves mega-portions, share the dish with someone else. Never be embarrassed to ask for a doggie bag. It's great to have the leftovers for another meal.

11. **Just say no to dessert—and if you can't, remember my four-bite rule.** To satisfy your sweet tooth, you can always order fresh fruit. Berries do it for me. If the pastry chef is a genius and you just can't resist, share a dessert or get a couple for the table to share. When a luscious, sinful confection is calling to you, go ahead and splurge, but don't eat the whole thing. Savor four bites—and enjoy each one to the max. You can offer what remains to your friends or family and let them consume the calorie bomb. Or you can ask your server to take it away. Whatever you do, don't take the rest home. If you're like me, you'll wake up in the middle of the night thinking of the treat in the refrigerator. Who needs a willpower struggle at 2 a.m.?

REAL TIME CHANGE

On most menus, there is a vegan/vegetarian option. Often I'd order a bunch of sides instead of a main dish—bean salad, steamed asparagus, fruit platter, and the like. While a bit pricey, I was able to eat out and enjoy my time with my family.

MICHELE BLOOM
SOUTH ORANGE, NEW JERSEY

ME: These are great strategies for not letting a menu get the best of you. You can find something to eat almost anywhere.

I enjoy conquering a menu. It's almost a game. Resisting the restaurant's best efforts to entice and seduce me is a challenge I have learned to rise to. I feel powerful and in control when I can enjoy a meal that is as good for me as it is delicious. My strategies for eating well anywhere are automatic now. If I indulge, it's because I choose to.

BEST BETS FROM AMERICA'S FAVORITE CUISINES

You know America is a melting pot when you consider how popular ethnic foods are. We are great fans of Italian, Chinese, Japanese, Mexican, Indian, and Thai foods. You can enjoy your favorite cuisines and still eat clean, whether you order takeout or go out. Here are some tips for healthy selections from around the world.

Italian Food

Italian food is so popular that it's practically not considered ethnic anymore. It's so much more than pasta and pizza. Italy is the home of the Mediterranean diet, which is as good as it gets. Mammoth portions of cheese-smothered pasta with meat served in Italian restaurants here would feed a table of six in Italy. You have to eat like an Italian for the healthiest meal.

- As always, get that breadbasket off the table. Focaccia is a killer. A single piece can have twice the calories as a piece of bread.
- You can construct a meal from antipasti: marinated or roasted vegetables, olives, artichokes, caponata, dried meats (like prosciutto, mortadella, and *bresaola*, which are very thinly sliced, so they are not that dangerous), grilled calamari, shrimp cocktail, giant fava beans, cannellini beans, garbanzo beans.
- Italian soups with combinations of escarole, beans, and sausage can be a meal. Minestrone, Italian wedding, and cioppino, a broth-based seafood stew, are my favorites.
- Many Italian restaurants are offering gluten-free pasta. Even so, don't eat the entire portion. Hollow pastas like ziti and orecchiette will make your portion look larger, so you will eat less. The opposite is true of

risotto, which is very dense. Stay away from the creamy, cheesy sauces and stick with tomato, pesto, and wine sauces. I like pasta made with just olive oil and garlic. Pasta primavera or pasta with clam sauce is always a good choice. If you can't resist the grated cheese, only use a little bit.

- You can always find grilled or roasted fish prepared with garlic, lemon, and olive oil and shellfish cooked in a broth for a main course. Avoid anything breaded or fried.

- Italians know how to make a great salad. Just make sure it isn't loaded with cheese.

- If you are only drinking one cup of coffee a day, save it for an espresso after your meal with a biscotti.

Chinese Food

Chinese cuisine is one of the most sophisticated in the world, but you wouldn't know that from the eggrolls and sesame noodles that top the list of American favorites. You can be more discriminating about what you order from a Chinese menu. Whether you are ordering takeout or attending a Chinese banquet, there are plenty of healthy foods to enjoy. Here are some general rules for eating Chinese food:

- Request that your meal be made without MSG, a flavor enhancer that can have side effects, including headaches, flushing, dizziness, intense thirst, sleepiness, or tingling in the mouth.

- Use chopsticks. You will eat less at a slower speed.

- Start with soup. Hot and sour or egg drop soup is a good choice.

- Request brown rice and eat like the Chinese: Use the dishes you've ordered as condiments for your rice.

- Focus on vegetables for appetizers. Order vegetable spring rolls rather than fried egg rolls. Lettuce wraps like chicken soong are delicious.

- Steamed anything is a good choice. Dumplings, vegetables, seafood, chicken, and meat are delicious when steamed. A whole steamed fish is a major treat.

- Chinese sauces can be full of salt, sugar, and fat. Ask for sauce on the side, or ask if your dish can be made with half the usual amount of sauce. Try to avoid soy sauce. Hoisin and plum sauce are good in a pinch.

Mexican Food

The fried tortilla chips, high-fat meats, sour cream, cheese, refried beans, and deep-fried combo plates that are part of most Mexican meals can be a mother lode of calories, fat, and sodium. You can sidestep these dishes and eat according to plan without much trouble. Mexican cuisine also has great salads, stews made of vegetables, and many great fish and chicken dishes. The cuisine is healthy by nature because it's about strong flavors like garlic, lime and citrus juice, oregano, and chili. Here are some suggestions for eating well at a Mexican restaurant.

- Resist the corn chips but save the salsa to use as a sauce.
- Skip the beer and save the margarita until the food is served.
- Ceviche is a protein-rich appetizer and a great way to start a meal. It consists of fresh raw fish, scallops, or shrimp marinated with diced vegetables and lime juice, which "cooks" the seafood.
- Order salads without the cheese and forget about the fried taco shell the salad arrives in.
- Ask for a side salad and toss it with salsa or guacamole.
- Order guacamole and use it instead of sour cream and cheese.
- Make sure the refried beans don't contain lard. Black beans and rice might be a better choice.
- Fajitas made with chicken, shrimp, or beef are a good option. You don't have to eat the soft tacos. Just say no to the tacos in advance.
- Chicken enchiladas without cheese can work. You can eat the filling and not the baked corn tortillas.
- Look for Veracruz sauce, which is made from tomatoes, onions, and chiles. In fact, dishes from the Mexican coast—Baja, the Yucatan, and Veracruz—tend to be lighter because they're beach food.
- Fish tacos are delicious—without the tacos.

- Mole sauce is divine. It's made from different nuts, seeds, spices, a number of peppers, and the best ingredient—Mexican chocolate. It's usually served with chicken.
- Tostadas have a pile of beans, meat, cheese, and salsa piled up on a flat taco shell. You can order a tostada without cheese and view the crispy corn taco as a plate.

Japanese Food

Japanese food has become very popular particularly with the diet-conscious. It's one of my favorite cuisines. Part of the appeal is that fish, vegetables, and rice are the main components of the Japanese diet and most dishes are prepared steamed, boiled, or raw. I can eat very clean, except for my lychee martinis, of course. That's not to say that you don't need some guidance when eating Japanese food. There are some things you need to know to order healthy.

- Choose a seaweed, cucumber, or house salad with ginger dressing on the side as your first course.
- Cold spinach with sesame is a good starter; steamed vegetable gyoza is another.
- Most Japanese sauces are loaded with salt. Ask for reduced-sodium soy sauce. If the dish you are ordering is sauced, ask for it on the side. Avoid mayonnaise-based sauces, which are used in spicy tuna roll, for example.
- Use wasabi, chili sauce, and ginger to season your food.
- Tempura is not the only fried food on the menu. Sushi rolls with "crunch" or "crunchy" in their description may mean an ingredient is fried.
- Ask for brown rice if it is available.
- Go with the classic rolls that have simple ingredients.
- Order vegetable rolls.
- Order salmon over tuna, because tuna is high in mercury.
- Try soba noodles, which are made of buckwheat.
- Stay away from sake. A 6-ounce serving of sake, which is liquid rice, is about 230 calories compared to 150 calories for an equal serving of wine.

- If your dish is sautéed, ask for it done lightly or with less oil.
- Use chopsticks to slow you down and to leave extra sauce at the bottom of the dish.

Indian Food

Menus at Indian restaurants are filled with dishes that are vegetable based or use lean cuts of meats, but there are land mines in the mix. Items like *palak paneer* and *malai kofta* are very rich—cooked with oil, butter, cream, and high-fat cheese. Here is some advice for ordering well.

- *Pappadams*, the wafer-thin disks brought to the table with sauces when you sit down, are made from chickpeas, rice flour, black gram, and lentils. They are either fried or cooked with dry heat. As long as they have not been fried, help yourself.
- Skip the fried appetizers such as samosas and *pakora*.
- Choose dishes made with lentils or chickpeas, such as dal or items labeled *chole*.
- Stick with chicken or seafood.
- Choose meats cooked tandoori style, which is oven grilled. Kebabs are always good.
- Stay away from dishes that include *paneer*, ghee, or *malai*. Paneer is similar to a full-fat cottage cheese, ghee is clarified butter, and malai is a cream used to make sauces.
- Eat veggie dishes like *aloo gobi* and *sukhi bhindi*.

Thai Food

Thai food is becoming more popular every day, because the flavors are bold and meld opposites: cooling coconut milk with fiery curry paste; sharp lime paired with musky fish sauce. The cuisine can be very rich, but there are many healthy things you can go for.

- Fish sauce, shrimp paste, and curry paste are very high in sodium, so if you have issues with blood pressure, cut back on your salt intake before eating Thai food.

- *Tom yum goong*, hot and sour shrimp soup, has a great balance of flavors and is a calorie bargain. Lean meat and mushrooms are simmered in broth with lemongrass, cilantro, and other seasoning.
- Stay away from the coconut soup—it's like a cream-based soup.
- Summer rolls are a delicious starter. Soft rice paper is wrapped around raw vegetables, rice noodles, shrimp, or a steamed filling. They are healthy, unfried egg rolls.
- *Satays* are grilled meat skewers. They are served with a peanut dipping sauce that you should go easy on.
- Papaya salad is crisply delicious. The grated fruit is in a chili lime dressing.
- *Larb* is a very spicy dish with coarsely chopped chicken, pork, or beef. Skip the pork.
- *Gai Pad Mamuang Him Ma Pahn* is cashew chicken—a winner.
- *Gaeng pah*, country-style curries, are made with water and are a good choice. They tend to be much spicier than coconut-based curries because there is no fat from coconut.
- Stay away from *massaman* curry, which is like the thick versions of curry made in India. It is cooked with potatoes, crushed peanuts, and coconut cream. Not for you.
- No sweet, sticky rice for you, either.

REAL TIME CHANGE

It takes a little effort, but it becomes easier to make the right choices when traveling and eating out. I try to stay prepared. When I travel, I bring a little lunch bag with avocados, nuts, almond butter, Mary's Gone Crackers, and goat Cheddar/brie so that I always have something delicious to eat when the appropriate choices are not available. Eventually, it becomes habit and not a bother or inconvenience.

LUCILLE IRCHA
NEW YORK, NEW YORK

ME: You've got this game beat. Once you have the right mind-set, it's easy to eat right anywhere. Veggie/protein, veggie/protein, veggie/protein—that's the key!

TAKING IT ON THE ROAD

When you're traveling, whether it's for business or pleasure, there is no reason to leave your new healthy eating habits behind. With a little bit of planning, you can avoid a minefield of dietary disasters. Begin by promising yourself that you will do your best to avoid fast food, even if you have clamoring kids. The familiarity of the fast-food chains might be easy and comforting in a strange place, but you are traveling to see the local culture. If you do find yourself at a restaurant with a mascot—never a good sign—order the healthiest food on the menu. It makes sense to do some research online before leaving. Check out the menus of local restaurants and the places to eat in your hotel. Then you won't be wandering around hungry looking for something to eat.

Whether you are flying, driving, or using another means of transportation, pack your own meal. It's easy enough to carry cut-up vegetables and a little container of hummus or a salad you made at home. I carry nuts, protein bars, fruit for snacks, and individual packets of nut butter during my travel time and on day trips during my vacation. Having snacks on hand during a day of sightseeing will keep the temptation to stop at the local bakery or ice-cream shop at bay. If you're a mother, you're used to carrying snacks for your children, so do the same for yourself.

If you are at the airport early, don't just sit at the gate waiting for your flight to be called. Stay active—you can window-shop. And never take a moving sidewalk at an airport. Burn up some energy instead.

Staying hydrated is especially important if you are flying. Low humidity and recirculating air in the cabin can dehydrate you, which will make you tired and make your jet lag worse. A good rule of thumb is to drink 8 ounces of water for every hour of the flight. While you are touring, you should always carry bottled water.

One of the best things you can do for yourself is to get rid of the key to the mini-bar. It's too tempting to raid it late at night. Stock your hotel room with bottled water, fresh fruit, and healthy snacks so you won't find yourself craving that giant, overpriced box of candy.

Forget late-night room service, too. If you're going to do room service, splurge on a healthy breakfast. Order breakfast the night before and schedule a wake-up call so that you have time to enjoy it. Having a good meal when you start the day will set you up for a full day of activities or business meetings. If your hotel offers a complimentary breakfast, go for protein, which will fill you up.

When you travel for business, bring workout clothes. If the hotel doesn't have a gym or an arrangement with a local gym, you can go for a brisk walk or run outside. If you are sightseeing, walk everywhere. Resorts and spas offer yoga and workout classes—take advantage of them. Most people say that they never gain weight when they travel. That's probably because they are more active than when they are at home.

You can observe the same guidelines for eating healthy that you do at home wherever you are. There is no reason to skip a special local dish, a festive cocktail, or a fabulous dessert—you're on vacation, after all. Keep portion control in mind. Moderation is the key. Sample new foods, don't feast on them. A treat a day is a good way to go. If you make a conscious choice to have that treat, you will enjoy the anticipation as well as the experience of eating it. Vacation is a time to unwind and restore yourself, to see new places and to try new things. You can do all that and still eat clean most of the time. It really isn't hard to do.

REAL TIME CHANGE

Not only do I feel better mentally as well as physically, I now realize that when I do have the occasional slipup, I can't beat myself up and let one mistake spiral into several, which is what I used to do. It's actually more motivating for me to get right back on the plan. . . . I am happy to know that I can enjoy my wine and desserts every once in a while and not get completely derailed from a life of eating well.

ELIZABETH BLOOM
NEW YORK, NEW YORK

ME: The problem is the next day. Don't keep walking on the wild side. You need to bring it back. Say, "No, it's not good for me." Now you are really in control. Recognizing that perfection isn't the goal makes the Clean Up Your Act Diet doable for the rest of your life.

WHEN YOU SLIP UP: THE MINI-CLEANSE

Even if you are careful about what you eat, remember that no one is perfect. You do not have to be pure all the time. You can indulge in a slice of birthday cake or a piece of fried chicken, but not every day. You have to make a conscious choice to go off plan. Be mindful of what you are doing. Don't slip into cheating. If you make an unhealthy choice, you have to be ready to compensate for it. If you have that cheeseburger on a brioche bun, eat very carefully for the next few days.

When you go off the rails and start to feel the effects of not eating mindfully, you can take steps to get back on track. I like to stop eating solid food for a day and have what I call a "blended salad" day. I make a puree of raw vegetables that is easily digested. The nutrients in the veggies are absorbed much more quickly than if I ate only salad for the day. A blended salad can look like green mush, but I like to think of it as green gazpacho. Just as it sounds, you put whatever you would eat in a salad into your blender and drink the puree. The soup is very healing and easy on your digestive track, which needs a rest if you've been bingeing. Blending the ingredients breaks down the cell walls of the vegetables, which releases the nutrition and chlorophyll. The puree still provides fiber, which you lose if you juice.

BLENDED SOUP

This soup is very refreshing. I play with different herbs to give it an extra kick. I've tried mint, parsley, tarragon, thyme—each has been great!

2 tomatoes

1 to 2 cucumbers, peeled

1/2 red bell pepper, seeds removed

Several leaves romaine, spinach, and/or other non-bitter greens

Scallions (optional)

2 ribs celery

1 clove garlic, peeled

1/2 to 1 avocado

1 tablespoon lemon juice or apple cider vinegar

Celtic sea salt

Fresh herbs

Put the tomatoes, cucumbers, pepper, greens, scallions (if using), celery, garlic, avocado, and lemon juice in a blender or food processor. Puree until smooth. Add the salt and herbs to taste. For a thinner soup, add filtered water gradually to reach the consistency you want.

Having a food-free day once in a while will keep you clean and stop any backsliding that might be going on. It's a good idea to schedule food-free days regularly. I try to do a day without chewing on the first Monday of every month—it keeps me honest!

REAL TIME CHANGE

I will do the cleanse every year. I see it as a refresher course. It'll get me to refocus, review what I should be doing, reinforce the good habits, and clean up the not-so-good ones. I think oftentimes we start off with the best of intentions, and then slowly we start to go back to our old ways, or at least some of them. So for me, not only will I do the cleanse again every couple of months, I'll review the Clean Up Your Act Diet, go over my notes, and reboot. That'll be a way of checking in to make sure I haven't been slipping—and if I have, then perhaps I can catch myself before I do too much damage. After all, I deserve it.

ILIANA GUIBERT
NEW YORK, NEW YORK

ME: I like the idea of repeating the cleanse annually as a refresher course. It's a good idea to reboot regularly.

STAY CLEAN WITH AN ANNUAL CLEANSE

I do the cleanse once a year, and Lisa does it twice. You should consider cleaning house annually, too. You've reduced the toxins that enter your body through the food you eat, and that's great. But the thousands of toxins that you can't avoid never take a holiday. You are constantly exposed to harmful chemicals that stress your body. You might be in good shape now, but who knows where you'll be a year from now. If some of the symptoms that went away while you were cleansing return, it's a signal from your body that you need help. If you start feeling creaky, bloated, or headachy, for example, don't wait a full year to deal with it. Make a correction right away. Every body is different. You have to learn to listen to yours, which will send you very clear signals. We all need a tune-up now and then. Toxic buildup doesn't stop completely once you eat clean.

I like to recapture the elation I feel once the cleanse kicks in. The experience

REAL TIME CHANGE

I will always do a cleanse annually. It was amazing. I cannot describe how almost immediately my insides felt better. I had every possible symptom during the cleanse, which proved to me it was working. I would never have believed how successful a cleanse could be until actually trying it myself.

LUCILLE IRCHA
NEW YORK, NEW YORK

ME: You'll know when it's time to do another cleanse. For me, the sign is when I start feeling a little off. You'll see. You become so used to feeling good that you'll be sensitive to when your liver needs a rest.

has been different every time. The cleanse seems to go deeper each time I do it, affecting so much more than my body. Cleansing gives me clarity and serenity, which are in short supply in life, as we know it today. Repeating the cleanse is also a reminder to make myself a priority and not to lose sight of my fundamental goal to be the best I can be every day.

Once you are off set meal plans, it might seem as if you are going to have to learn how to cook all over again. You just need to shift your focus a bit. From a quick roasted chicken to a berry tart, from pizza to biscotti, the recipes in the next chapter will show you that you don't have to give up your favorite foods to stay on the Clean Up Your Act Plan.

I've learned that people will forget what you said, people will forget what you did, but people will never forget how you made them feel.
—MAYA ANGELOU

CHAPTER

10

No-Fuss Recipes

STARTERS

SOUPS

MAINS

VEGGIE BURGERS

PIZZAS

SIDES

DESSERTS

I love to cook for friends and family—the more the merrier. I started a tradition when we lived in Snedens Landing. I had fabulous parties for the cast of *The Sopranos* every season. I'd set up little candlelit tables outside overlooking the Hudson. Fifty of us would feast and have a great time. We were serenaded by Dominic Chianese playing his guitar. Now, when I'm in Bridgehampton, I have a regular Monday night dinner for my friends, who are more than welcome to bring their friends. The number keeps growing, and I need a bit of help, but I'm in there putting it all together.

There is something about a home-cooked meal that brings people together in a relaxed way. Food was important in my family. My English mother, who wasn't the best cook, learned family recipes from my Italian grandmother. Holiday meals were unforgettable, and I like to carry on the tradition. Margaux and her husband, Deric, are excellent cooks. When my friend and his boys drop off striped bass they catch off Montauk, Deric marinates and grills it to perfection. You can't get fresher fish than that! One time last summer, they caught so much that I was able to feed 30 people!

I read cookbooks and food magazines the way some people read novels. I know my way around a kitchen and like to throw things together. For me, simple food is the best food. My palette has definitely changed since I cleaned up my act. I don't need fancy sauces and elaborate recipes. The food I enjoy most is fresh and pure.

In putting together the recipes for this chapter, I wanted to give you a range—from quick, basic recipes to more sophisticated combinations. A number of the recipes were inspired by recipes I found on the Web sites of the *New York Times,* Martha Stewart, and Oprah, but I've adapted them to my own tastes and dietary requirements. I included a number of recipes that put quinoa to good use to give you an idea of how versatile that super grain is. Desserts can be a challenge if you are eating gluten free, sugar free, and dairy free, so there are a number of simple recipes that will satisfy your sweet tooth. Baking is an ambitious undertaking, but it's doable. You'll find good recipes for tart and pie crusts, which you can fill as you'd like. If you are a baker, you'll want to check out cookbooks for gluten-free baking. The good news is that you can find substitutions now for everything you need for success.

As you experiment with cooking for your new way of eating, I hope you'll share your recipes with us by posting them on my Web site, tothefullestbook.com. I'm always ready to try something new.

STARTERS

HUMMUS

MAKES 6 SERVINGS

Fresh homemade hummus is quick and easy and tastes so much better than store bought. Hummus is high in fiber that slows digestion and keeps blood sugar levels from rising too quickly. The chickpeas in hummus are a complete protein, a healthy source of carbohydrates, and contain iron and manganese, which keep up energy levels. Tahini, made from sesame seeds, is high in protein and a great source of calcium. The garlic and olive oil are good for you, too. In place of mayo or butter, I use hummus to "butter" my wraps and as a dip for anything. You can store hummus in an airtight container for a week in the refrigerator. Here is a basic recipe along with ideas for variations.

$\frac{1}{4}$ cup tahini

$\frac{1}{4}$ cup fresh lemon juice (about 1 large lemon)

1 clove garlic, minced

3 tablespoons extra virgin olive oil, divided

$\frac{1}{2}$ teaspoon ground cumin

$\frac{1}{2}$ to 1 teaspoon Celtic sea salt

1 15-ounce can chickpeas (garbanzo beans)

2 to 3 tablespoons water

Dash of paprika

1. In the bowl of a food processor, combine the tahini and lemon juice. Process for 1 minute. Scrape the sides and bottom of the bowl, then process for 30 seconds to whip or cream the tahini.

2. Add the garlic, 2 tablespoons of the oil, cumin, and salt. Process for 30 seconds.

3. Drain and rinse the chickpeas with water.

4. Add half the chickpeas to the food processor and process for 1 minute. Scrape the sides and bottom of the bowl, add the remaining chickpeas, and process for 1 to 2 minutes. If the hummus is too thick or still has tiny bits of chickpea, slowly add the water while the processor is turned on, until the consistency is perfect.

5. Scrape the hummus into a bowl. Drizzle the remaining 1 tablespoon oil over the top and sprinkle with the paprika.

(continued)

VARIATIONS:

Garlic hummus: Add 3 garlic cloves to the processor.

Red pepper hummus: Add ½ cup roasted red bell peppers to the processor.

Artichoke hummus: Add 1 can drained artichoke hearts to the processor.

Roasted or sun-dried tomato hummus: Add 3 tablespoons roasted tomatoes or sun-dried tomatoes with a bit of fresh parsley or basil.

Beet hummus: Boil 2 red beets in water until tender, then chop and toss them into the food processor along with the hummus and extra tahini, lemon juice, and oil.

Spicy black bean hummus: Use equal parts hummus and black beans with some jalapeño pepper, cilantro leaves, and lime juice.

Olive hummus: Add ¼ cup chopped olives—green with pimiento or kalamata olives—and a dash of cayenne pepper.

Lemon-ginger hummus: Add the juice of another lemon to the hummus and a 1-inch piece of ginger, peeled and minced.

Pine nuts, parsley, and lemon juice hummus: Toast ¼ cup pine nuts in a dry skillet, then stir into the hummus with a little lemon juice and chopped parsley. Save some of the nuts to sprinkle on top with a little olive oil.

I could go on and on—the possibilities are limitless. Make sure you have cans of chickpeas and tahini in your pantry. You will get great at creating your own combinations.

Mango Salsa

MAKES 6 SERVINGS

Mangoes are so good for you, and they have so much flavor. I use this salsa on chicken, fish, eggs, wraps, and gluten-free crackers.

2 ripe mangoes, peeled, seeded, and chopped

1 red onion, chopped

1 bunch cilantro, stemmed and chopped

1 lime

1. In a bowl, combine the mangoes, onion, and cilantro.

2. Squeeze the juice from the lime onto the mixture and mix well.

3. Cover and refrigerate for 1 hour.

Mushroom Pâté

MAKES 8 TO 10 SERVINGS

This rich vegetarian pâté has a nutty flavor. I sometimes use it in wraps or with raw veggies and gluten-free crackers. My guests always love it.

1 tablespoon extra virgin olive oil

½ cup chopped onions

1 clove garlic, minced

2 cups white mushrooms, thinly sliced

½ teaspoon dried savory or fresh herbs of your choice

Celtic sea salt and freshly ground black pepper

½ cup raw cashews

Fresh parsley, chopped, for garnish

1. In a large skillet, heat the oil over medium heat. Add the onion and garlic, cover, and cook for 5 minutes, or until softened.

2. Add the mushrooms and savory. Add salt and pepper to taste. Cook uncovered, stirring occasionally, for 5 minutes, or until the mushrooms are soft and the liquid is evaporated.

3. In a bowl of a food processor, grind the cashews to a fine powder. Add the cooled mushroom mixture to the bowl and process until smooth.

4. Spoon the pâté into a small crock or serving bowl. Smooth the top and sprinkle with the parsley.

5. Cover and refrigerate for at least 1 hour before serving.

WHITE BEAN PUREE

MAKES 6 SERVINGS

Lucille Ircha, a corporate flight attendant and one of the Rodale test panelists, prepares food served on private jets. She gave us this simple recipe for pureeing beans. In the morning, she eats the puree with eggs, but this versatile recipe can be used as a dip served with gluten-free crackers or raw veggies or as a side with steamed veggies. You can use any kind of organic canned beans, but white beans are her favorite.

1 15-ounce can organic white beans

3 cloves garlic

½ cup pitted olives

2 tablespoons extra virgin olive oil

¼ cup fresh lemon juice (about 1 large lemon)

1 teaspoon dried oregano

Celtic sea salt and freshly ground black pepper

Paprika for garnish

1. In a food processor or blender, combine the beans, garlic, olives, oil, lemon juice, oregano, salt, and pepper. Process until smooth.

2. Place in a bowl and sprinkle with paprika.

SOUPS

SIMPLE CHICKEN SOUP

MAKES 6 TO 8 SERVINGS

This recipe is as basic as it can be. It's the soup Lisa made for me the first time I did the cleanse. If you'd like, you can add a cup of cooked quinoa or some steamed vegetables. I sometimes add parsnips, dill, and parsley.

1 3½- to 4-pound chicken

6 carrots, peeled

4 ribs celery

1 large yellow onion

1½ teaspoons Celtic sea salt

1 teaspoon whole black peppercorns

1. Place the chicken in a large pot.

2. Cut 3 of the carrots and 2 of the celery ribs into 1-inch pieces. Quarter the onion.

3. Add the cut vegetables to the pot with the salt, peppercorns, and enough cold water to cover (about 8 cups). Bring to a boil. Reduce the heat and simmer, skimming any foam that rises to the top, for 30 minutes, or until the chicken is cooked through.

4. Transfer the chicken to a bowl and let cool.

5. Strain the broth, discarding the vegetables. Return the broth to the pot.

6. Thinly slice the remaining 3 carrots and 2 celery ribs. Add them to the broth and simmer for 10 minutes, or until tender.

7. When the chicken is cool enough to handle, shred the meat and add it to the soup.

BLACK BEAN SOUP

This hearty soup really sticks to your ribs. I serve it with chopped onions, tomatoes, and avocados. You can use a dollop of this thick, tasty soup to spice up a wrap.

1 tablespoon olive oil

1 medium onion, chopped

12 cloves garlic, minced

2 teaspoons chili powder

1 teaspoon ground cumin

2 15-ounce cans organic black beans, rinsed and drained

1¾ cups organic vegetable broth

½ cup chopped cilantro

1 lime, cut into wedges

1 avocado, sliced (optional)

1. In a 3-quart pot, heat the oil over medium heat. Add the onion and garlic and cook until tender.

2. Stir in the chili powder, cumin, beans, and broth, and heat to boiling. Reduce the heat to low and simmer for 15 minutes.

3. Use a blender, food processor, or mixer to blend the soup to a creamy consistency.

4. Serve garnished with the cilantro, lime wedges, and avocado slices, if using.

MULTITASKING VEGETABLE SOUP

MAKES 4 TO 6 SERVINGS

This is a delicious, hearty soup that is very versatile. I get many meals out of it. I take out some vegetables with a slotted spoon and serve them over brown rice or quinoa as a stew. I add a shredded chicken breast, some rotisserie chicken, or a piece of firm fish like haddock. I even use the vegetables in an omelet.

2 tablespoons olive oil

½ small onion, thinly sliced

1 rib celery, thinly sliced

1 large carrot, thinly sliced

1 medium parsnip, thinly sliced

2 cloves garlic, diced

2 leeks, thinly sliced

1 cup chopped kale

1 cup chopped collard greens

1 cup shredded cabbage

1½ cups tomatoes, diced, with juice

2 15-ounce cans organic great Northern beans (or any kind)

1 quart vegetable broth or water

1 teaspoon dried thyme

1 bay leaf

1. In a large Dutch oven or stockpot, heat the oil over medium-high heat. Add the onion, celery, carrot, parsnip, garlic, and leeks and sauté until soft.

2. Add the kale, collard greens, and cabbage and stir to coat. Reduce the heat to low and cover the pot. Cook for 3 minutes, or until the greens are wilted and soft.

3. Add the tomatoes and beans. Increase the heat and bring to a simmer.

4. Add the broth and bring back to a simmer. Add the thyme and bay leaf. Simmer for at least 30 minutes.

5. For the best flavor, remove the soup from the heat and let sit for 1 hour, covered, before serving. It can be reheated.

MAINS

MY SLOW COOKER BEEF STEW

There's nothing like a slow cooker to make your life easy. I have found that the order you put the ingredients in makes a difference, so add the ingredients as listed. I make a lot of this stew because it freezes well.

2 pounds cubed beef

Gluten-free flour

Grapeseed or olive oil

1 bottle robust red wine, such as cabernet sauvignon

3 beef bouillon cubes

2 medium onions, chopped

4 ribs celery, cut into $\frac{1}{2}$-inch slices

3 carrots, cut into $\frac{1}{2}$-inch slices

3 parsnips, cut into $\frac{1}{2}$-inch slices

2 turnips, peeled and cut into 1-inch cubes

At least 8 cloves garlic

$\frac{1}{2}$ head cabbage, sliced

3 tablespoons tomato paste

1. Dredge the beef in the flour and brown in the oil.

2. Put the browned beef in a stockpot and cover with water.

3. Pour in the wine and add the bouillon cubes. Add the onions, celery, carrots, parsnips, turnips, garlic, and cabbage. Add the tomato paste and stir lightly.

4. Cook on high for 4 to 5 hours or on low for 8 hours.

ROASTED LEMON CHICKEN

MAKES 6 SERVINGS

I love this recipe. I make two chickens at a time so that I always have chicken ready to eat as a snack or for a meal.

½ cup Dijon mustard

¼ cup low-sodium tamari

¼ cup lemon juice (about 1 large lemon; save the rinds)

1 4½- to 5-pound chicken

3 lemons

Mix of fresh herbs: rosemary, sage, thyme, parsley, and oregano—or you can just use one herb

Cracked black pepper

1. Preheat the oven to 425°F.

2. Make the marinade by placing the mustard, tamari, and lemon juice in a bowl and whisk until the ingredients are well blended into a smooth, creamy consistency.

3. Clean the chicken well and pat dry. Place in a roasting pan or baking dish. Stuff the cavities with the lemon rinds and fresh herbs.

4. Pour the marinade over the chicken. Sprinkle the pepper and some more of the herbs, chopped, on top of the chicken.

5. Cover with aluminum foil and place on the lower rack of the oven.

6. Bake for 1½ hours, then remove the foil. Baste with the pan juices. Roast, basting every 15 minutes, until a meat thermometer reads 180°F.

QUICK ROASTED CHICKEN

MAKES 4 TO 6 SERVINGS

This is a perfect recipe, inspired by a classic from Marcella Hazan, a great Italian cook. It has become so popular in the past three decades that everyone roasts chicken this way. I use this simple recipe when I am in a rush. It makes a scrumptious chicken every time.

1 2½-pound broiler chicken

Salt and freshly ground black pepper

2 lemons

Hot sauce (optional)

1. Preheat the oven to 350°F.

2. Wash the chicken inside and out. Pat dry with a paper towel.

3. Sprinkle the salt and pepper inside and out, and rub into the surfaces with your fingertips.

4. Wash the lemons and soften them by pressing them between your palms and rolling them back and forth a few times. Pierce the lemons with a fork and place them inside the chicken. You can close the opening of the chicken with toothpicks if you like, but it's not necessary.

5. Sprinkle some hot sauce on the skin, if using.

6. Put the chicken in a roasting pan and place in the upper third of the oven. Roast for 25 minutes. Increase the heat to 400°F and roast for 15 minutes. If you're lucky, the skin puffs up.

STUFFED PEPPERS

MAKES 8 SERVINGS

I often freeze a few cooked stuffed peppers and pop them into the oven when I don't feel like cooking. All I need to do is make a tossed salad and I have a great meal.

4 bell peppers, any color

2 cups cooked quinoa or brown rice

1 15-ounce can organic stewed tomatoes

1 small onion, chopped

1 cup chopped fresh mushrooms

1 tablespoon minced fresh basil

Salt and freshly ground black pepper

1. Preheat the oven to 350°F.

2. Cut the bell peppers in half horizontally and place in an oven-safe dish.

3. Mix together the quinoa, tomatoes, onion, mushrooms, basil, and salt and black pepper to taste.

4. Stuff the pepper halves with the mixture.

5. Bake for 30 minutes.

WINTER SQUASH AND BEAN STEW

This meat-free stew really fills you up. It's best to make this a day ahead for richer flavor. I've adapted the recipe to use organic canned beans rather than cooking the beans from scratch, to cut back on preparation time.

> 4 15-ounce cans organic pinto beans with liquid
>
> 1 tablespoon extra virgin olive oil
>
> 1 onion, chopped
>
> 1 tablespoon sweet paprika
>
> 4 large cloves garlic, minced
>
> 1 14-ounce can chopped organic tomatoes with liquid
>
> $\frac{1}{2}$ teaspoon Celtic sea salt
>
> 1 bay leaf
>
> 1 pound butternut squash, peeled and cut into $\frac{3}{4}$-inch cubes
>
> 1 cup water
>
> 1 cup quinoa, rinsed
>
> Freshly ground black pepper

1. Place the beans and their liquid in a large pot and heat over medium heat.

2. In a large nonstick skillet, heat the oil over medium heat and add the onion. Cook, stirring, for 5 minutes and then add the paprika. Stir for 1 minute.

3. Add the garlic and stir for 2 more minutes.

4. Stir in the tomatoes and salt. Cook, stirring, for 5 to 10 minutes, or until the tomatoes have cooked down slightly.

5. Remove from the heat and scrape the mixture into the pot of beans.

6. Bring the beans to a simmer and add the bay leaf and squash. Simmer, covered, for 30 minutes, or until the squash and beans are tender.

7. Add the water and quinoa. Simmer for 20 to 30 minutes. Add a little more water if it is absorbed quickly.

8. Add the pepper and more salt to taste and simmer for 2 more minutes.

QUICK CHERRY TOMATO SAUCE

This recipe is great for the tomatoes I grow in my garden—that is, if there are any left after I eat them sun-warmed off the vine! I've estimated the measurements for the ingredients, because I eyeball this sauce. You'll get the hang of it. The sauce is great on chicken, quinoa, brown rice or quinoa pasta, and spaghetti squash as suggested in the cleanse menu.

3 tablespoons extra virgin olive oil

3 cloves garlic, crushed

$\frac{1}{2}$ cup diced eggplant, bell peppers, onions, summer squash, or anchovies (for flavor), or a mixture of any of these ingredients

1 pint cherry tomatoes, halved

Salt and freshly ground black pepper

1 tablespoon dried rosemary or oregano

Basil or parsley for garnish

1. In a 10- or 11-inch skillet, heat the oil and garlic gently over low heat, letting the garlic soften but not brown.

2. Increase the heat, add the vegetables and cook until soft.

3. Add the tomatoes, salt and pepper to taste, and the rosemary or oregano. Increase the heat and simmer for 15 to 20 minutes, or until the sauce is thick and pulpy.

4. Remove from the heat and stir in the basil or parsley.

Vegetable Frittata with Quinoa

MAKES 6 SERVINGS

You can do so much with eggs—I eat them all the time. I just throw anything that I have in the fridge into the frittata. Feel free to substitute your favorite vegetables: spinach, mushrooms, and cauliflower are always delicious. When I have guests for breakfast, I'll prepare the frittatas in advance and warm them up or serve at room temperature. That way, I'm not stuck in the kitchen scrambling or flipping. Frittatas work for lunch and dinner, too.

2 cups organic vegetable stock

1 cup diced parsnips

1 cup broccoli florets

1 cup sliced zucchini

1 cup quinoa, rinsed

½ cup diced plum tomatoes or canned organic diced tomatoes

2 teaspoons herbes de Provence (sage, oregano, marjoram, basil, and thyme in equal parts)

2 teaspoons goat cheese

4 eggs

1 teaspoon soy-free butter substitute (optional) or extra virgin olive oil

1. Preheat the oven to 375°F.

2. In a large saucepan over medium heat, bring the stock to a boil. Add the parsnips and cook for 5 to 7 minutes. Remove the parsnips with a slotted spoon and place in a large bowl.

3. Add the broccoli to the stock and cook for 5 to 7 minutes. Remove with a slotted spoon and add to the bowl with the parsnips.

4. Add the zucchini to the stock and cook for 1 minute. Remove with a slotted spoon and add to the same bowl.

5. Add the quinoa to the stock, bring to a boil, and cook for 5 minutes. Remove the quinoa with a slotted spoon and add to the same bowl. The remaining broth can be used later as a base for soup, or freeze it in ice cube trays for use in cooking.

6. Add the tomatoes, herbes de Provence, and goat cheese to the bowl with the vegetables and quinoa. Mix until the cheese combines with the other ingredients.

7. In a small bowl, whisk the eggs. Add to the vegetable mixture and stir gently.

8. Heat the butter substitute (if using) or the oil in a 10-inch nonstick ovenproof skillet over medium heat. When the butter is frothy or the oil is hot, reduce the heat to medium-low and add the frittata mixture. Cook for a few minutes, then finish in the oven until done to your taste. (Note that the fritatta will continue to cook after it's removed from the oven.) Remove from the oven.

9. Hold a plate upside down on top of the skillet and flip the two over together. You can brush the top of the frittata with melted butter substitute or olive oil and serve with gluten-free toast.

MEDITERRANEAN LETTUCE WRAPS

MAKES 4 SERVINGS

I live on wraps—there are so many combinations. This one is fresh, light, and satisfying. You can use rice noodle wraps or a slice of turkey or roast beef, if you prefer.

1 avocado, chopped

$\frac{1}{2}$ cup finely chopped scallions

$\frac{1}{2}$ small cucumber, cubed

3 tablespoons sliced black olives

1 small red bell pepper, thinly sliced

2 tablespoons goat or sheep yogurt

2 large tomatoes, sliced

2 teaspoons lime juice

Freshly ground black pepper

4 large leaves romaine lettuce

1. In a large salad bowl, toss together the avocado, scallions, cucumber, olives, bell pepper, yogurt, tomatoes, lime juice, and black pepper.

2. Place a lettuce leaf on each plate and scoop some of the salad mixture onto it.

3. Roll the lettuce, turning in the ends, so the salad does not fall out.

ROASTED BRUSSELS SPROUTS, MUSHROOMS, AND PINE NUTS WITH GREMOLATA ON A BED OF QUINOA

MAKES 4 TO 6 SERVINGS

Roasted Brussels sprouts are at the top of my list. Gremolata—a combination of garlic, parsley, and lemon juice—is a simple, classic Italian sauce with flavor that can't be beat. It makes anything taste delicious.

1 pound Brussels sprouts, trimmed and cut in half

⅓ cup pine nuts

1 pound mushrooms, halved or quartered depending on size

Celtic sea salt and freshly ground black pepper

3 tablespoons extra virgin olive oil

2 cloves garlic, finely minced

¼ cup finely minced flat-leaf parsley

2 teaspoons finely chopped lemon zest

3 cups cooked quinoa

Crumbled feta or goat cheese

1. Preheat the oven to 425°F. Line 2 baking sheets with parchment paper and brush with olive oil.

2. Place the Brussels sprouts and pine nuts on one baking sheet and the mushrooms on the other. Sprinkle with salt and pepper. Drizzle 1½ tablespoons of the oil over each.

3. Place both sheets in the oven and roast for 20 minutes, stirring halfway through. When done, the Brussels sprouts will be browned on the edges and tender. The mushrooms will be soft and there will be juice on the baking sheet.

4. Meanwhile, make the gremolata by mixing together the garlic, parsley, and lemon zest in a small bowl.

5. In a large bowl, place the mushrooms with the juice and the Brussels sprouts mixture. Pour in the gremolata and toss together.

6. Spoon the quinoa onto plates and top with the vegetables and any remaining juice in the bowl.

7. Crumble the cheese on top and serve.

VEGGIE BURGERS

I'm a meat lover, but I'm always on the lookout for great veggie burgers. So many prepared veggie burgers contain soy and corn—GMO no-nos. I like fooling around with recipes and have come up with many variations. Make a big batch of veggie burgers and freeze what you don't eat. A well-stocked freezer can help you stay on track effortlessly.

GREENS AND QUINOA BURGERS

MAKES 4 TO 6 SERVINGS

I'm always looking for ways to eat more greens, and quinoa has become one of my favorite ingredients. I keep a supply of these in the freezer ready to eat. These burgers are great!

½ to ¾ pound beet greens, Swiss chard, spinach, or kale or any combination of greens

2 cups cooked quinoa

2 to 3 tablespoons extra virgin olive oil, divided

⅔ cup finely chopped carrots

⅔ cup finely chopped onions

2 teaspoons minced fresh ginger

Celtic sea salt

1 teaspoon cumin seeds, toasted and crushed

2 cloves garlic

1 15-ounce can organic chickpeas (garbanzo beans) or kidney beans

2 tablespoons fresh lemon juice

1 egg

Freshly ground black pepper

1. Preheat the oven to 375°F.

2. Steam the greens for 2 minutes above boiling water. Transfer to a bowl of cold water, drain, and squeeze out the excess water.

3. Chop the greens medium fine and place in a large bowl. Add the quinoa and combine well.

(continued)

4. Heat 1 tablespoon of the oil in a medium skillet over medium heat. Add the carrots and onions. Cook for 3 minutes, or until tender.

5. Add the ginger and a pinch of salt. Cook for 3 minutes, or until the vegetables are tender.

6. Add the cumin and garlic and stir for 1 minute.

7. Remove from the heat and stir into the greens and quinoa mixture.

8. In a food processor or blender, puree the chickpeas, lemon juice, and egg.

9. Stir into the bowl with the greens and quinoa. Add salt and pepper to taste.

10. With wet hands, form the mixture into 4 to 6 patties.

11. Heat an ovenproof skillet and add 1 tablespoon of the oil. Cook the patties for 1 to 2 minutes, or until browned. Flip them and put the skillet in the oven.

12. Bake for 10 to 15 minutes, or until browned. If the patties fall apart, use a spatula to press them together.

VEGGIE BURGERS WITH NUTS

MAKES 4 SERVINGS

This is a flavorful veggie burger. You can make it simply or spice it up. Either way, or in any combination, it's delicious! I love this with slices of avocado.

1 cup hazelnuts or Brazil nuts, or ½ cup of each

½ cup coarsely chopped onions

½ cup coarsely chopped celery

½ cup coarsely chopped carrots

½ cup fresh cilantro leaves

¼ cup sesame seeds

½ teaspoon Celtic sea salt

½ teaspoon dried dill

1 egg

½ teaspoon ground cumin (optional)

½ teaspoon ground coriander (optional)

1. Preheat the oven to 400°F. Line a baking sheet with parchment paper and coat with olive oil cooking spray.

2. In a food processor, combine the nuts, onions, celery, carrots, cilantro, sesame seeds, and salt. Process for 20 to 30 seconds.

3. Add the dill, egg, and cumin and coriander, if using. Process for 10 seconds, or until well mixed.

4. Spoon 4 mounds of the mixture onto the baking sheet. Use a rubber spatula to flatten and shape into round patties.

5. Bake for 15 to 20 minutes, or until golden brown. Remove from the oven and let stand for a few minutes before serving.

RAINBOW BURGERS

MAKES 10 SERVINGS

Quinoa, sweet potatoes, spinach, and red lentils make a very colorful burger. These tasty burgers are packed with healthy ingredients and look great on the plate. You can serve them with mango chutney and tomato slices. Served with a salad, these burgers make a great meal.

$\frac{1}{3}$ cup quinoa, rinsed

$\frac{1}{3}$ cup red lentils, rinsed

$1\frac{2}{3}$ cups water

$\frac{1}{2}$ teaspoon Celtic sea salt

$1\frac{1}{2}$ pounds sweet potatoes, baked

3 cups chopped and tightly packed fresh spinach

$\frac{3}{4}$ cup crumbled feta

3 tablespoons chopped fresh mint

$\frac{1}{4}$ cup minced chives

2 teaspoons fresh lemon juice

Freshly ground black pepper

1 cup chickpea flour

$\frac{1}{4}$ cup extra virgin olive oil, divided

1. Put the quinoa, lentils, water, and salt in a saucepan and bring to a boil. Reduce the heat, cover, and simmer for 15 to 20 minutes, until the quinoa and the lentils are tender.

2. Drain any water remaining in the saucepan through a strainer and return the quinoa and lentils to the pan. Cover the pot with a towel, then cover with a lid and let sit for 15 minutes.

3. Skin the baked sweet potatoes and put the pulp in a large bowl. Mash them with a fork.

4. Add the spinach and mash together using your hands, if you wish. Add the quinoa and lentils, feta, mint, chives, lemon juice, and salt and pepper to taste. Mix well. The mixture should be moist.

5. Form $\frac{1}{3}$ cup of the mixture into a ball. Try wetting your hands to reduce sticking. Roll the ball in the flour, then gently flatten into a patty. Set on a plate and continue with the rest of the mixture. Refrigerate uncovered for at least 1 hour.

6. Prepare for the cooked burgers by placing a rack over a sheet pan.

7. Heat 2 tablespoons of the oil in a 12-inch heavy nonstick skillet over high heat. Swirl the pan to coat with the oil. Lower the heat to medium and place 4 to 5 patties in the pan. Do not crowd. Cook for 4 minutes, or until well browned on one side.

8. Turn and brown for 4 minutes. Remove to the rack.

9. Heat the remaining 2 tablespoons oil in the skillet and cook the remaining patties. Place on the rack.

10. Keep the patties warm in a low oven until ready to serve.

Advance preparation: You can form the patties and keep them refrigerated for up to 2 days, or cook them all the way through and keep them refrigerated for 2 or 3 days. They also freeze well, cooked or uncooked. Thaw completely before reheating. To reheat cooked patties, place on a baking sheet in a low oven for 10 to 15 minutes.

PIZZAS

Bet you thought you'd never eat pizza again without guilt! You might not be eating a slice from your corner pizzeria, but there are endless variations you can make that are healthy and sophisticated. I've included a simple recipe for a good gluten-free pizza crust. Some grocery stores are selling ready-made or frozen gluten-free pizza dough. Boxed gluten-free pizza dough mixes are also available. See what you can find and keep some in your freezer or pantry. You can use goat cheese mozzarella and Manchego, a sheep cheese from Spain that melts well. Halloumi, a grilling cheese from Cyprus made from goat's and sheep's milk, has become very popular. It has a strong flavor but works well on veggie pizzas. I've given you a number of pizzas to give you an idea of how much you can do on a crust. It's as varied as making a sandwich. You have to break out of the sauce-cheese-and-pepperoni habit.

GLUTEN-FREE PIZZA CRUST

MAKES 2 (12-INCH) CRUSTS

This recipe is simple and freezes well. Once you have the dough on hand, you can put dinner on the table in a half hour. You can make the dough in advance. It will keep in the refrigerator for a few days and will stay fine in the freezer for up to 3 months.

2 cups all-purpose gluten-free flour

$1\frac{1}{2}$ teaspoons xanthan gum

1 tablespoon active dry yeast

1 teaspoon granulated stevia

$\frac{3}{4}$ teaspoon coarse Celtic sea salt

3 tablespoons extra virgin olive oil plus extra for drizzling

$\frac{3}{4}$ cup warm water

1. Put the flour, xanthan gum, yeast, stevia, and salt in a bowl or a food processor. If you are working by hand, stir constantly while streaming first the oil, then the water, until the mixture begins to come together. If using a food processor, pulse while streaming the oil and water until a ball begins to form. If the dough appears sticky, add more flour a tablespoon at a time.

2. Press the dough into a disk.

3. Place the dough in a bowl and drizzle with the oil. Turn the dough to coat with oil, which will prevent a crust from forming while it rises. Cover the bowl with plastic wrap and place in a warm, draft-free area to rise for 1 hour, or until it is double in size.

4. After the dough has risen, wrap in plastic wrap and chill for 1 hour before rolling out.

5. Preheat the oven to 400°F.

6. Divide the dough into 2 balls. Roll out each ball between two sheets of parchment or waxed paper. Roll in the edges and brush the dough with oil.

7. Bake for 5 to 7 minutes.

8. Place the toppings on the crust and return to the oven. Bake until the ingredients are cooked and the cheese is melted.

To freeze for later use: Just after the dough has risen, put it into a plastic freezer bag. Take it out of the freezer in the morning and bake it for dinner that night.

Grilled Artichoke, Sweet Pepper, and Mushroom Pizza

MAKES 6 SERVINGS

This is an example of a pizza you can make on a prebaked crust and then finish on a grill. You can throw just about anything on the crust, and it will be a treat.

1 prebaked 12-inch gluten-free pizza crust (see Gluten-Free Pizza Crust on page 206)

½ teaspoon extra virgin olive oil

⅔ cup organic sugar-free tomato sauce

2 plum tomatoes, sliced

¼ cup chopped bell pepper

¼ cup sliced fresh mushrooms

¼ cup chopped water-packed artichoke hearts, drained and rinsed

2 tablespoons sliced ripe olives

1 cup shredded goat mozzarella cheese

½ cup crumbled feta cheese

1½ teaspoons minced fresh basil or ½ teaspoon dried

1½ teaspoons minced fresh rosemary or ½ teaspoon dried

1½ teaspoons minced chives

1. Preheat the grill.

2. Brush the crust with the oil. Spread the tomato sauce over the crust to within 1 inch of the edges.

3. Top with the tomatoes, bell pepper, mushrooms, artichokes, and olives. Sprinkle the cheeses on top.

4. Grill the pizza, covered, over medium indirect heat for 12 to 15 minutes, or until the cheese is melted and the crust is lightly browned.

5. Sprinkle with the basil, rosemary, and chives the last 5 minutes of cooking.

6. Let stand for 5 minutes before slicing.

VARIATION:

If you do not want to grill this, preheat the oven to 400°F (or whatever the package requires if you are using store-bought dough). Put the pizza on a pizza stone or parchment-covered upside-down baking sheet and bake for 15 minutes.

Pizza a la Grecque with Halloumi Cheese

MAKES 4 SERVINGS

Eating this pizza makes me feel as if I'm in Greece. Using traditional Greek ingredients on a pizza is a nice twist.

2 tablespoons olive oil, divided

1 cup cherry tomatoes

1 clove garlic, coarsely chopped

Coarse Celtic sea salt and freshly ground black pepper

Gluten-free flour

Gluten-free pizza dough (see Gluten-Free Pizza Crust on page 206)

1 cup grated halloumi cheese

2 tablespoons pine nuts

2 cups baby arugula

1 tablespoon red wine vinegar

¼ cup coarsely chopped kalamata olives

1. Preheat the oven to 450°F. Rub a baking sheet with oil.

2. In a food processor, combine 1 tablespoon of the oil, the tomatoes, garlic, salt, and pepper. Pulse three or four times, until ingredients are chunky. Set aside.

3. On a work surface lightly dusted with gluten-free flour, use a rolling pin and your hands to roll and stretch the dough until it is large enough to cover the surface of the baking sheet. Let the dough rest if it becomes too elastic. Transfer to the baking sheet.

4. Spread the reserved tomato sauce over the dough, leaving a 1-inch border all around.

5. Top with the cheese and pine nuts. Season to taste with salt and pepper.

6. Bake for 15 to 20 minutes, or until the crust is golden.

7. In a medium bowl, toss the arugula with vinegar, the remaining 1 tablespoon oil, and salt and pepper to taste.

8. Sprinkle the arugula mixture and olives over the pizza.

Spring Medley Pizza

MAKES 4 SERVINGS

I'm crazy about artichokes, and this is a very satisfying combination of flavors. The pie looks great, too!

> 1 12-ounce jar marinated artichoke hearts, drained well, reserving the marinade; artichokes quartered if whole
>
> 1 pound asparagus, trimmed, cut into 2-inch pieces, and halved lengthwise if thick
>
> 1 pint yellow, orange, and red cherry or grape tomatoes, halved
>
> 1 pound gluten-free pizza dough, halved (see Gluten-Free Pizza Crust on page 206)
>
> Coarse Celtic sea salt and freshly ground black pepper
>
> 7 ounces grated Manchego or mozzarella goat cheese

1. Preheat the oven to 500°F. Move the racks to the upper and lower thirds of the oven.

2. In a large bowl, combine the artichoke hearts, asparagus, and tomatoes.

3. Place the dough halves on a large piece of parchment paper. Brush one half with the marinade from the artichoke hearts and roll out to a 14-inch oval.

4. Transfer the dough and the parchment paper to a rimmed baking sheet.

5. Top with half the vegetable mixture, leaving a 1-inch border, and season with salt and pepper. Brush the border with the marinade.

6. Repeat to make a second pizza.

7. Bake both for 10 minutes, rotating the sheets halfway through. Sprinkle the pizzas evenly with the cheese and bake for 3 to 5 minutes, or until the crust is golden and the cheese is melted.

GRILLED CALIFORNIA VEGETABLE PIZZA

MAKES 4 SERVINGS

A salad never tasted so good! This is a great summer pizza. Avocado on pizza reminds me of California.

3 tablespoons olive oil, divided

Gluten-free flour

1 pound gluten-free pizza dough (see Gluten-Free Pizza Crust on page 206)

2 plum tomatoes, thinly sliced crosswise

2 scallions, white and green parts separated, thinly sliced

1 5-ounce log soft goat cheese, crumbled

Coarse Celtic sea salt and fresh ground black pepper

1 5-ounce bag organic baby spinach

1 avocado, diced

2 tablespoons red wine vinegar

1. Preheat the grill to medium. Brush a large rimless baking sheet with 1 tablespoon of the oil.

2. On a surface lightly dusted with gluten-free flour, roll and stretch the dough to two 8-inch ovals or rounds. Transfer to the prepared sheet.

3. Brush the tops with 1 tablespoon of the oil.

4. Transfer the dough to the grill and cook for 2 to 3 minutes, or until the undersides are firm and begin to char. Use tongs and a large spatula to flip the crusts onto a baking sheet, grilled side up.

5. Place the tomatoes, scallion whites, and cheese on the crusts. Season with salt and pepper.

6. Slide the pizzas back onto the grill. Cook for 3 to 5 minutes, rotating occasionally, until cooked through and the cheese begins to melt. Transfer to a cutting board.

7. In a medium bowl, combine the spinach, avocado, scallion greens, vinegar, and the remaining 1 tablespoon oil. Season with salt and pepper and toss to combine. Arrange evenly onto both pizzas, then halve and serve.

SIDES

I am going to call these recipes side dishes, but I eat each and every one as a main course or a snack. I am totally fluid about what I eat when. I have included some basic recipes as well as some that are more creative to show you how much you can do with healthy food.

ROASTED VEGGIES

Crunchy roasted vegetables are a delicious side dish and snack. I eat bowls of them during the day. I love Brussels sprouts, broccoli, carrots, parsnips, eggplant, cauliflower, green beans, halved cherry tomatoes or tiny plum tomatoes, onions, and butternut squash done this way. If you roast kale, you have kale chips! Yum. Sometimes I mix the vegetables for a colorful snack. You can combine roasted vegetables with quinoa for a balanced meal. Experiment with the seasoning. I like to use cumin on carrots and basil and garlic with the tomatoes.

1. Preheat the oven to 350°F. Line a baking sheet with parchment paper to save on cleanup time.

2. Prepare the vegetables as if you were going to steam them—by cutting them into bite-size pieces. Put them in a plastic bag, add a little extra virgin olive oil (not too much), and shake to coat.

3. Spread them in a single layer on the baking sheet. Season with salt.

4. Bake for 25 to 45 minutes, depending on how crisp you want your veggies and the size of the pieces. Smaller pieces cook quickly.

VEGETABLE QUINOA

Quinoa is such a nutritious grain, and it's so versatile. And it's a satisfying substitute for rice and pasta. I can't get enough of it. Try this basic recipe, then create your own delicious combinations of your favorite vegetables. Be creative—you can use any kind of raw, sautéed, or roasted vegetables. Greens are especially delicious.

1 medium red onion

4 ribs celery

2 carrots

2 tablespoons olive oil, divided (1 tablespoon is optional)

1 cup quinoa, rinsed

2 cups water or low-sodium vegetable stock

4 cloves garlic

Salt and freshly ground black pepper

Parsley or cilantro, for garnish

1. Roughly chop the onion, celery, and carrots. Set aside if leaving raw. For less crunch, sauté with 1 tablespoon olive oil in a medium saucepan over medium-low heat for 5 minutes, or until tender.

2. Add the quinoa and the water or stock to a medium pot. Add the garlic, 1 tablespoon oil, and salt and pepper to taste.

3. Bring to a boil. Reduce the heat to low and simmer for 15 minutes, or until all the liquid is absorbed by the quinoa.

4. Add the vegetables.

5. Serve garnished with parsley or cilantro.

VARIATION AFTER THE CLEANSE:

Add ½ cup cubed goat or feta cheese.

Hot Lentil Salad

This is a delicious dish that I eat cold, too. Lentils are nutritious and easy to make. You do not have to soak them overnight, and they cook quickly. Cooked lentils will keep refrigerated for about a week. Any amount of lentils can be cooked as described below. Just maintain the 2:1 ratio of water to lentils. Season them with olive oil, lemon juice, vinegar, and fresh herbs, and eat them on their own. Lentils can also be added to soups, salads, or other recipes.

1 cup brown or green lentils

2 cups water

1 bay leaf

¼ teaspoon salt

4 tablespoons extra virgin olive oil

1 onion, chopped

4 ribs celery, sliced

2 cloves garlic, crushed

2 zucchini, diced

¾ cup green beans, cut into short lengths

½ red bell pepper, diced

½ yellow bell pepper, diced

1 teaspoon Dijon mustard

1 tablespoon balsamic vinegar

Freshly ground black pepper

1. Measure the lentils into a strainer or colander. Pick over and remove any shriveled lentils, debris, or rocks. Thoroughly rinse under running water.

2. Transfer the lentils to a saucepan and pour in the water. Add the bay leaf. Bring the water to a rapid simmer over medium-high heat, then reduce the heat to maintain a very gentle simmer. You should only see a few small bubbles and some slight movement in the lentils.

3. Cook, uncovered, for 20 to 30 minutes. Add water as needed to make sure the lentils are just barely covered. Lentils are cooked as soon as they are tender and no longer crunchy. Older lentils may take longer to cook and shed their outer skins as they cook.

4. Strain the lentils and remove the bay leaf. Return the lentils to the pan and stir in the salt.

5. Meanwhile, heat the oil in a large skillet and add the onion, celery, garlic, zucchini, and green beans. Cook for 5 minutes.

6. Add the bell peppers to the skillet and cook for 1 minute.

7. Stir in the mustard and vinegar.

8. Pour over the cooked lentils and toss. Season to taste with salt and black pepper.

QUINOA TABBOULEH

MAKES 8 SERVINGS

Tabbouleh is one of my favorite side dishes. Replacing couscous with quinoa makes this tabbouleh nuttier and more nutritious.

1 cup white quinoa, rinsed

1 cup organic vegetable broth

½ cup grated carrots

1 rib celery, chopped

1 cup diced tomatoes

1 cup diced cucumber

1 cup chopped fresh parsley

DRESSING

⅛ cup olive oil

¼ cup fresh lemon juice (about 1 large lemon)

2 tablespoons minced garlic

2 tablespoons chopped fresh mint

Celtic sea salt and freshly ground black pepper

1. Put the quinoa in a saucepan, add the broth, and bring to a boil. Reduce the heat to low and simmer for 12 minutes, or until the broth is absorbed.

2. In a large bowl, stir together the carrots, celery, tomatoes, and cucumber. Add the quinoa and parsley and combine.

3. *To make the dressing:* In a container with a lid, combine the oil, lemon juice, garlic, mint, salt, and pepper. Shake to mix.

4. Pour the dressing over the quinoa mixture and toss well. Season to taste with salt and pepper.

DESSERTS

The one thing people seem to miss the most on the Clean Up Your Act Diet is a sinful dessert. If you need a break from fresh fruit, a little ingenuity will fulfill your cravings. Remember, even if you are following the program and avoiding gluten, dairy, and sugar, you still have to be mindful of how much dessert you eat. It should not be a daily event.

In adapting your recipes, you should know a bit about how to substitute stevia, which is on the plan, for sugar. Stevia is significantly sweeter than sugar so you don't have to use very much. Granulated stevia is now available—Stevia in the Raw, Pure Via, and NuNaturals Stevia Baking Blend are good products. In this form, stevia has a 1:1 ratio with sugar, so you use the same amount of stevia as you would sugar. This chart should help you figure it out.

CONVERTING SUGAR TO STEVIA

SUGAR	GRANULATED STEVIA	STEVIA PACKETS	STEVIA BULK	CLEAR STEVIA LIQUID
1 tsp	1 tsp	½ packet	¼ tsp	⅛ tsp
2 tsp	2 tsp	1 packet	½ tsp	¼ tsp
¼ cup	¼ cup	6 packets	3 tsp	½ tsp
⅓ cup	⅓ cup	8 packets	4 tsp	¾ tsp
½ cup	½ cup	12 packets	6 tsp	1¼ tsp
¾ cup	¾ cup	18 packets	9 tsp	1¾ tsp
1 cup	1 cup	24 packets	12 tsp	2½ tsp
2 cups	2 cups	48 packets	24 tsp	5¼ tsp

I don't want to overwhelm you, but if you use honey or maple syrup as a sweetener, you have to use less than if you were using sugar. The general rule is:

1 cup sugar = ¾ cup maple syrup
1 cup sugar = ½ cup honey
More than 1 cup sugar = ⅔ to ¾ of the honey, depending on desired sweetness

You can do the math!

Gluten-Free Vanilla Almond Biscotti

MAKES 10 TO 12

You should see me in the kitchen making big trays of biscotti for the holidays. It's so much fun, and everybody loves them. This recipe works well on the plan.

1½ cups gluten-free flour

½ teaspoon xanthan gum

1 teaspoon baking powder

¼ teaspoon kosher salt

½ cup granulated stevia

¾ cup raw almonds, finely chopped

2 large eggs

2 tablespoons soy-free butter substitute, melted

2 teaspoons vanilla extract

1 teaspoon almond extract

1. Preheat the oven to 350°F. Place a piece of parchment paper on a rimmed baking sheet.

2. In a large bowl, add the flour, xanthan gum, baking powder, salt, and stevia and whisk to combine. Stir in the almonds. Add the eggs, butter substitute, vanilla, and almond extract and mix. The texture of the batter should be like cookie dough but not too sticky. If necessary, knead the dough with wet hands until smooth.

3. Place the dough in the center of the baking sheet and shape a loaf that is about 7 inches long x 3 inches wide x 1 inch thick.

4. Place in the center of the oven and bake for 20 minutes, or until golden brown and firm.

5. Remove from the oven and allow to cool for at least 10 minutes.

6. Lower the oven temperature to 300°F.

7. Slice the loaf at a 45-degree angle into 10 to 12 biscotti about ¼ inch thick.

8. Spread the biscotti about 1 inch apart on the baking sheet and bake for 10 minutes. Flip them over and bake for 10 minutes if you want crunchy cookies, less if you want softer ones.

9. Remove from the oven and allow to cool to room temperature. The cookies will get crisp as they cool.

Note: You can store biscotti at room temperature in an airtight container for 2 days. If you're freezing biscotti, wrap it and place in a freezer-safe container.

GLUTEN-FREE CHOCOLATE ALMOND BISCOTTI

MAKES 20

This is a different take on biscotti. The chocolate and vanilla biscotti look so good together on a platter.

2 tablespoons soy-free butter substitute, melted

⅓ cup maple syrup

½ teaspoon almond extract

2 eggs

1 cup almond meal

1½ cups gluten-free flour

½ teaspoon xanthan gum

1 teaspoon baking powder

Pinch of Celtic sea salt

3 tablespoons cocoa powder

½ cup slivered almonds

1. Preheat the oven to 300°F. Place a piece of parchment paper on a baking sheet.

2. In a large bowl, add the butter substitute, maple syrup, almond extract, and eggs and mix with a hand mixer. Add the almond meal, flour, xanthan gum, baking powder, salt, cocoa powder, and almonds and mix. The texture of the batter should be like cookie dough but not too sticky. It has to be malleable enough to knead.

3. Divide the dough in half and create 2 logs about 12 inches long x 3 inches wide x 1 inch high.

4. Place on the baking sheet. Bake for 25 minutes.

5. Remove from the oven and let cool for 10 minutes.

6. Cut the logs at a 45-degree angle to get about 10 biscotti per log.

7. Spread the biscotti on the baking sheet and bake for 10 minutes. Flip them over and bake for 10 minutes.

Vanilla Chia Seed Pudding

MAKES 4 SERVINGS

When you have a dessert craving, chia seed pudding will fill the bill. The gelling characteristic of the chia seeds makes this like tapioca pudding. It's delicious and filled with important nutrients.

$\frac{1}{4}$ cup raw chia seeds

2 cups unsweetened almond milk

$1\frac{1}{4}$ teaspoons vanilla extract

1 tablespoon maple syrup (optional)

Pinch of Celtic sea salt

1. Put the chia seeds in a medium bowl.

2. Add the almond milk, vanilla, maple syrup (if using), and salt and whisk to combine.

3. Cover the bowl with plastic wrap and let sit for 30 minutes. Then refrigerate for at least 4 hours. Letting the pudding rest overnight is the best way to go.

TOPPINGS:

Be creative here. Some of the combos I like are:

Cinnamon and almonds

Strawberries and almonds

Mixed berries with lemon zest

Watermelon with mint

Sliced bananas and cinnamon

Dark chocolate shavings

Mango and coconut

CHOCOLATE CHIA SEED PUDDING

This variation will make you chocoholics happy. If you have a chocolate craving, you can satisfy it with a nutritious treat.

1¼ cups unsweetened almond milk or coconut milk

¼ cup chia seeds

3 tablespoons raw cacao powder (baking cacao also works)

Dash of Celtic sea salt

1 tablespoon maple syrup (optional)

Dark chocolate shavings for garnish

1. In a medium bowl, mix the milk, chia seeds, cacao powder, salt, and maple syrup, if using.

2. Cover tightly with plastic wrap. Refrigerate at least 4 hours or overnight.

3. Serve garnished with dark chocolate shavings.

TOPPINGS:

Shaved 70 percent chocolate

Shaved ginger

Strawberries and almonds

Raspberries and coconut

Sliced bananas

Melon and mint

Coconut

CRUMBLES

If you love pies, crumbles are a gluten-free solution. You can use any seasonal fruit and create a perfect dessert. I keep a supply of the topping in the freezer in case I come home from the farmers' market and am inspired to throw a crumble together. This topping does the trick.

THE CRUMBLE TOPPING

MAKES ENOUGH FOR 1 CRUMBLE

1¼ cups gluten-free rolled oats

½ cup quinoa flour

⅓ cup granulated stevia

½ teaspoon freshly grated nutmeg

½ teaspoon cinnamon

⅛ teaspoon Celtic sea salt

6 tablespoons cold, unsalted soy-free butter replacement (you can find sticks), cut into ½-inch pieces

1. Preheat the oven to 350°F. Cover a baking sheet with parchment paper.

2. In a food processor, place the oats, flour, stevia, nutmeg, cinnamon, and salt. Pulse several times to combine.

3. Add the butter substitute and pulse until the butter is evenly distributed through the grain mix. The consistency should be crumbly.

4. Spread the topping on the baking sheet.

5. Bake for 10 minutes. Rotate the pan front to back, stir the mixture, and bake for 5 to 10 minutes, or until browned.

Note: This topping will keep in the freezer for several weeks in a freezer bag or airtight container.

MAKING A CRUMBLE

What follows are general directions for constructing a crumble.

1. Preheat the oven to 350°F. Use soy-free butter substitute to butter a 2-quart baking dish.

2. Scrape whatever fruit mixture is used and all of the juice in the bowl into the baking dish.

3. Put the baking dish on a baking sheet so that it is easy to handle and place it in the oven. Bake 20 to 25 minutes, or until the fruit is bubbling and the liquid is syrupy. Allow to cool if desired.

4. About 30 minutes before serving, spread the crumble topping evenly over the fruit mix. Bake for 20 minutes, until the topping is nicely browned.

5. Remove from the heat and cool for 10 minutes before serving.

There is nothing like a home-baked dessert—and this is so little trouble! Here are a few fruit combos for your crumbles. The possibilities are limitless.

MIXED FRUIT CRUMBLE

MAKES 8 SERVINGS

This crumble is as colorful as it is delicious.

2½ pounds peaches or nectarines, sliced

1 cup blueberries, raspberries, blackberries, or a mix of berries

2 tablespoons maple syrup

½ teaspoon ground cinnamon

1 teaspoon vanilla extract

1 teaspoon almond extract

PLUM AND FIG CRUMBLE

MAKES 8 SERVINGS

This is a sophisticated and surprising combination that seems as if it should take more effort than it does. I love recipes like that!

2 pounds red-fleshed plums, pitted and cut into sixths

6 fresh figs, stemmed and cut in half

1 tablespoon granulated stevia

½ teaspoon ground cinnamon

1 tablespoon plum brandy or red wine (optional)

1 teaspoon arrowroot

PEAR AND GINGER CRUMBLE

MAKES 8 SERVINGS

This crumble has a little kick. The mild pear gets a boost from the ginger.

3 pounds pears (about 5 large ones), peeled, cored, and sliced

1 tablespoon + 1 teaspoon maple syrup

1 tablespoon fresh lemon juice

2 tablespoons chopped candied ginger

½ teaspoon vanilla extract or the seeds from ½ vanilla bean

2 teaspoons arrowroot

APPLE CRUMBLE

I couldn't leave out an apple crumble. I love to get apples at an orchard in the fall and make this crumble. Apples dry out in the oven, so the baking instructions for this crumble are different from the other crumble recipes.

$2\frac{1}{2}$ pounds thinly sliced apples

2 tablespoons granulated stevia

1 tablespoon fresh lemon juice

$\frac{1}{2}$ teaspoon ground cinnamon

$\frac{1}{4}$ teaspoon ground nutmeg

1 teaspoon vanilla extract

$\frac{1}{3}$ chopped walnuts (optional)

1. Preheat the oven to 375°F.

2. Follow the general directions, but bake the apple and walnut mixture for 30 minutes, stirring every 10 minutes, or until the apples are tender.

3. After topping the apples with the crumble, bake for 15 to 20 minutes.

ICE POPS

Ice pops for grown-ups are all the rage. They are so refreshing on a summer day and satisfy my sweet tooth anytime. You can find the plastic molds in just about any housewares store or department—or just use paper cups with Popsicle sticks.

PEACH AND HONEY POPS

MAKES 6 TO 8

This recipe puts peaches to good use—and the color is beautiful.

4 ripe peaches
¼ cup honey
1 tablespoon fresh lemon juice

1. Bring a large pot of water to a boil. Cut an X on the bottom of the peaches.

2. Place the peaches in the boiling water for 1 to 2 minutes, or until the skins start to pull away.

3. Transfer the peaches to a strainer and rinse under cold running water for a minute or two. Slip off the skins.

4. Cut the peaches into chunks and mash well in a large bowl.

5. Add the honey and lemon juice to the bowl and mix well.

6. Pour the mixture into molds and insert the sticks. If using cups, freeze for 30 minutes until slushy, then insert the sticks.

7. Freeze for at least 6 hours.

TEA AND POM POPS

This is an unusually refreshing combination!

2 cups water

2 hibiscus tea bags

$\frac{1}{3}$ cup granulated stevia

$\frac{2}{3}$ cup pomegranate juice

1 tablespoon lemon juice

1. Bring the water to a boil in a saucepan.

2. Add the tea bags and let stand for 5 minutes.

3. Remove the tea bags and discard.

4. Whisk in the stevia. Pour into a bowl and let cool.

5. Stir in the pomegranate and lemon juice.

6. Pour the mixture into molds and insert the sticks. If using cups, freeze until slushy and then insert the sticks.

7. Freeze for at least 6 hours.

MELON-LIME POPS

This pop satisfies a sugar craving every time.

$\frac{1}{4}$ cup water

$\frac{1}{4}$ cup granulated stevia

1 ripe honeydew (about $3\frac{1}{2}$ pounds), peeled, seeded, and cut into $\frac{1}{2}$-inch pieces (4 cups)

$\frac{2}{3}$ cup fresh lime juice

1. Heat the water in a small saucepan and stir in the stevia to dissolve. Let cool.

2. In a blender, place half of the melon and half of the lime juice. Blend until smooth.

3. Add the stevia syrup and the remaining melon and lime juice. Puree until smooth.

(continued)

4. Force the puree through a fine-meshed sieve into a bowl. Press on the solids and then discard them.

5. Pour the mixture into molds and insert the sticks. If using cups, freeze for 30 minutes until slushy, then insert the sticks.

6. Freeze for at least 6 hours.

RASPBERRY-WATERMELON POPS

MAKES 6 TO 8

I can't wait for my granddaughter, Vivienne, to be old enough to eat one of these pops!

3 cups watermelon cubes

2 cups fresh or frozen raspberries

¼ cup granulated stevia

1 tablespoon lime juice

1. In a blender, combine the watermelon, raspberries, stevia, and lime juice. Puree until smooth.

2. Push the mixture through a fine strainer with a flexible spatula and discard the solids.

3. Pour the mixture into molds and insert the sticks. If using cups, freeze for 30 minutes until slushy, then insert the sticks.

4. Freeze for at least 6 hours.

Almond Meal Pie or Tart Crust

This crust is great with fruit tarts or pies that only require a bottom crust. I love the texture, and the added nuttiness is delicious. I thought I'd include this basic recipe to solve the gluten-free crust dilemma. You can experiment with fillings.

2 cups almond meal

$\frac{1}{3}$ cup arrowroot

1 teaspoon baking powder

$\frac{1}{2}$ teaspoon xanthan gum

1 teaspoon Celtic sea salt

$\frac{1}{3}$ cup cold soy-free butter substitute

$\frac{1}{3}$ cup water

1. Preheat the oven to 350°F.

2. In a large bowl, combine the almond meal and arrowroot. Add the baking powder, xanthan gum, and salt and mix well.

3. Add the butter substitute a little at a time and mix with a fork or pastry cutter until the mixture is crumbly.

4. Add the water slowly until the mixture forms a ball.

5. Divide into 2 balls. Cover and chill for at least 30 minutes.

6. Roll out each ball between 2 sheets of waxed paper. The dough tears easily, so be careful when you transfer it to a pie dish or tart pan.

7. If you are not adding filling before baking, prick the bottom of the crust with a fork to avoid bubbles.

8. Bake for 30 minutes after you add the pie filling.

PARISIAN BERRY AND CUSTARD TART

This beautiful tart will prove that you can cook just about anything and stick to the Clean Up Your Act Plan. It's a winner that will please everyone.

CRUST

2 cups gluten-free flour, sifted

1½ cups granulated stevia or sugar substitute

¼ cup chilled soy-free butter substitute, cut in small pieces

2 egg yolks

2 tablespoons ice water

CUSTARD

2 cups rice or almond milk

3 eggs, lightly whisked

1 teaspoon vanilla extract

¼ cup granulated sugar substitute

½ to 1 cup mixed berries

1. *To make the crust:* Preheat the oven to 350°F.

2. In a food processor, combine the flour, stevia or sugar substitute, and butter substitute. Pulse until the mix looks like fine bread crumbs. Add the egg yolks and water. Process until the dough just starts to come together.

3. Press the dough into a ball and knead until almost smooth. Do not overwork the dough. Wrap it in plastic wrap and refrigerate for 30 minutes.

4. Place between 2 sheets of floured parchment paper. Roll out to a 12-inch disc.

5. Place in a 10-inch fluted tart pan with a removable base. Trim the excess. Lightly prick the bottom with a fork. Return it to the refrigerator for 15 minutes.

6. Cover the pastry with parchment paper and fill with pastry weight, rice, or beans.

7. Bake for 10 minutes. Remove the paper and weights. Bake for 10 minutes. Remove and lower the oven temperature to 300°F.

8. *To make the custard:* Place the milk in a saucepan and bring to a simmer over low heat.

9. In a bowl, whisk the eggs, vanilla, and sugar substitute. Whisk in the hot milk. Strain through a sieve. Pour into the cooked pastry.

10. Bake for 30 minutes, or until just set. Remove from the oven and let cool.

11. Top with the mixed berries or mixed fruit laid out in a nice pattern.

I'm not a Le Cordon Bleu chef, but I don't want to eat that way—at least not all the time. The recipes in this chapter are wholesome and easy to prepare. Since you want to eat as much fresh food as possible, I wanted to show you how easy and satisfying it can be to eat healthy with just a little planning. Let us know if you come up with twists and variations on these recipes.

You need to support your good eating habits with exercise to deepen your transformation. Moderate exercise is an excellent preventive action to take against age-related illness. If you want to age gracefully, you have to keep moving. You need to burn energy to create more. You will find a sane plan to get you going in the next chapter.

I resolve to go down fighting.
—LORRAINE BRACCO

CHAPTER

11

Moving Is Huge

Not much will age you as quickly as being sedentary. You've got to keep moving if you want to stay healthy and energetic. You have to burn energy to feel more energetic. Our muscles shrink as we age, and the loss of muscle mass means sagging, droopy skin, because muscles prop up the skin. Increased muscle tone and elasticity will keep you looking fit and vital. Even better, muscle tissue burns more calories than fat, so building muscles helps to keep your weight under control. Weight-bearing exercise will also protect you from weakened, fragile bones. Regular exercise reduces the harmful effects of stress on your body, increases circulation, improves sleep, and builds muscle mass. Exercise will keep you flexible—no more creaking joints—preserve your balance, and improve your posture. Being active will not only make you look and feel better, but your take on life will be more optimistic. Exercise alleviates depression and anxiety and will boost your sense of well-being. Doesn't all this make you want to get moving?

REAL TIME CHANGE

I feel my mood has changed. I used to feel down all the time, and now I feel more like myself before all the weight gain. I have more energy, too, and that has enabled me to exercise more often. I have regained the energy I thought was gone forever.

ANA NAPOLES
BLOOMFIELD, NEW JERSEY

ME: When you fuel your body with healthy food, you have so much more energy. Burning energy through exercise defuses stress, which goes a long way to making you feel more upbeat and rejuvenated.

Making moderate exercise an essential part of your life starts now. The good news is that going from an inactive lifestyle to a moderately active one produces the greatest health improvements. One of the fundamental changes in your life from this day on has to involve moving more. I am not talking about torturing yourself. I am definitely not a fitness fanatic. I won't do a workout so tough that I can't walk the next day. I hate pain! I want to feel limber, toned, and strong, and I know from experience that the only way to achieve that is to get regular exercise. I've found what works for me. I am addicted to Pilates. The slow movements release tension in my muscles and make me feel lengthened. Aside from walking a lot, I take a Pilates class on the reformer three times a week. I love that there are women in their eighties in the class doing Pilates with kids who are 23. Pilates is terrific. It stretches me out and makes my core strong. It's not a complete snap, but it's not excruciating in any way. I have to confess that I moan and groan my way through the workout to the amusement of the others in the class.

You don't want to overdo it when you are on your 14-day cleanse. Your body will be busy cleaning itself from the inside out. Forget about doing an intense workout, a long-distance run, an uphill bike ride, or a Zumba class during the 2 weeks of your cleanse. Treat yourself gently while you are detoxing. Your aim is to get out all the kinks and feel good in your body. But that doesn't mean you should become a couch potato. You don't have to kill yourself—you just have to get your blood moving.

Here are some suggestions for Days 1 and 2 of the cleanse, when you might feel a bit tired.

- Stretch when you get out of bed in the morning. Reach high for the ceiling with both arms, arch your back, fold over and touch your toes—even if you have to bend your knees. Do this in a relaxed way. Do not push too hard. Get the kinks out of your body.
- Try to take a 10-minute walk around the block after every meal. Get outside, breathe in the air, and enjoy the world around you.

AFTER THE FAST DAYS

You should work up to doing 30 minutes of moderate exercise three or four times a week. You do not have to work out with a trainer until your muscles ache and you're paralyzed the next day. There are so many choices out there.

When I'm vacuuming or tidying up, I play music and move. I love to dance and make my house a regular dance club. Housework has never been so much fun! When Lisa comes to visit, we dance and laugh our heads off. Don't be surprised if you see me on the "Happy" 24-hour dance videos on YouTube.

The secret is to find something you enjoy doing. You might like to ride a bike, practice yoga, or take your dog on long walks. My dog, Elsie, is such a happy camper now! You could swim, play tennis, ski, or join a gym with a wide selection of classes that interest you, from Zumba to yoga. You could have a trainer design a simple weight program for you at the gym, or buy some light hand weights to use at home while you are watching TV. If you have a stationary bike or treadmill that is collecting dust or serving as a clothing rack, clear the equipment off and use it. Listening to music, the radio, or watching old movies while you walk or ride at a moderate pace will make the time fly. There are also TV channels dedicated to exercise. Check them out. It's like having a personal trainer on call anytime. There are DVDs available on everything from Pilates Mat Exercises to yoga to aerobic dancing. It's a good way to try different kinds of exercise programs. It's fine to change it up, as long as you get some exercise most days of the week.

If you are starting from zero, work your way up to the equivalent of 30 minutes of exercise a day. Start with a relaxed walk after each meal. Don't even time it. Then build up to two 10-minute walks a day and increase your pace. Once you are walking at 30 minutes at a clip, add on Pilates, yoga, weight training, or any combination of physical activities a couple of times a week. It won't take long before you won't feel right unless you move. Daily exercise should be like brushing your teeth.

The young woman who gives me manicures was constantly complaining about her weight. When she saw how I had changed, she asked me what she should do. I told her to stop drinking soda and to park her car far from the shop. It didn't take long before those small changes began to make a difference in how she looked and felt. She started adding more physical activity to her life. Since she was losing weight and inches, she was motivated to change how she ate. I'm away for several weeks at a time, so I notice how much she has changed each time I see her. She's so much happier and looks fabulous now that she is transforming herself.

REAL TIME CHANGE

I have been walking to work instead of taking the subway from Penn Station. When time is short, I get off the subway one or two stops early and walk the rest of the way. My family has started a new tradition of walking in the park after dinner. While more of a stroll than a power walk, I am up and moving nonetheless.

MICHELE BLOOM
SOUTH ORANGE, NEW JERSEY

ME: What a terrific family tradition! It's wonderful that you are making movement a way to bring your family closer. Once you get into the habit of walking after a meal, it'll change your whole body. And turning your commute into an opportunity to move more is such a good use of your time.

There are countless opportunities to build movement into your life. Don't park your car close to where you are headed. Instead, find the parking space that is farthest away. Take the stairs rather than the escalator or elevator. You've heard tips like this before—put them into action now. Here are other painless ways to incorporate more movement into your life.

- Multitask—take a walk when you talk with a friend on the phone, do squats or leg lifts as you brush your teeth, balance on one foot as you comb your hair, pace during business calls, listen to an audiobook when you walk.
- Stand at your desk—you will burn more calories. In fact, sitting for 9 hours a day or more is lethal. Get up and move.
- Walk for part of your lunch break, or select a restaurant that's not too close to the office.
- Meet a friend for coffee and go for a walk carrying your coffee cups.
- Stand on public transportation.
- Take a stroll around the office once a day.
- Don't use drive-through windows—park and get out of your car to get your coffee or do your banking.
- Put away your TV remote and get up to change channels.
- Carry your groceries to your car instead of using the cart.
- Use a restroom on a different floor and take the stairs.
- Walk to a colleague's office instead of calling.
- Spend time playing with children.
- Clean and sweep vigorously.
- Ride a bike or walk to do chores.

REAL TIME CHANGE

My daughter, who is a personal trainer and has "coached me" with proper posture for the plan, says she has noticed a slight change in the fit of my clothes. I made a conscious effort to move whenever possible. I jumped rope, stretched, walked, and made extra physical activity during work hours.

HELYN L. BRYANT
HILLCREST, NEW YORK

ME: Lucky you to have a personal trainer in the family. Make sure she teaches you and helps you to make movement a part of your life.

- Plant a garden, rake leaves, or weed.
- Get off a bus or subway a stop early.
- Do calf raises while you're standing on line.
- Stretch or do a weight routine during commercials.
- Take up a new sport or activity like tennis, hiking, golf, or ballroom dancing.

THE 30-DAY PLANK CHALLENGE

I picked up this static exercise from Gilles Baudin, a trainer in the Hamptons. It is a one-stop workout that will send your core strength through the roof. You don't need special equipment or clothing. All you have to do is hold a position—nothing else. It looks easy, but it isn't! Remember, this is a beginner routine. Everyone starts somewhere. Do the best you can and enjoy the challenge.

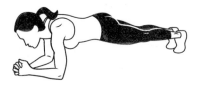

THE PLANK

Lie on your stomach. Raise your upper body with your forearms on the floor and push up from your toes. Hold your body in a straight line. That's all there is to it.

What I love about this exercise is that you can do it anywhere—in your office, a hotel room, or in front of the TV. Though the plank exercise may seem like nothing, it has many benefits and targets an area of the body that needs attention as we age. This exercise:

- Strengthens your lower back
- Develops your core muscles—the abs, back, hips, and butt
- Develops your abdominal muscles by targeting the rectus abdominals, also known as the abs and lower abs—often a problem area

The idea is that over a period of 30 days you increase the amount of time you hold this position. Go up in increments of 5 seconds and make sure you have a rest day once each week. If you get stuck at any length of time, stay there until it is easy and you are ready to move on.

Here is a plan.

Day 1: 15 seconds	**Day 16:** 45 seconds
Day 2: 15 seconds	**Day 17:** 45 seconds
Day 3: 20 seconds	**Day 18:** 50 seconds
Day 4: 20 seconds	**Day 19:** Rest
Day 5: 20 seconds	**Day 20:** 50 seconds
Day 6: Rest	**Day 21:** 50 seconds
Day 7: 25 seconds	**Day 22:** 55 seconds
Day 8: 25 seconds	**Day 23:** 55 seconds
Day 9: 25 seconds	**Day 24:** 1 minute
Day 10: 30 seconds	**Day 25:** 1 minute
Day 11: 30 seconds	**Day 26:** Rest
Day 12: 35 seconds	**Day 27:** 1 minute 10 seconds
Day 13: Rest	**Day 28:** 1 minute 20 seconds
Day 14: 40 seconds	**Day 29:** 1 minute 30 seconds
Day 15: 40 seconds	**Day 30:** Plank for as long as possible

THREE SIMPLE ROUTINES TO RAISE YOUR LEVEL OF FITNESS

Whether you never leave your couch if you can help it, try to stay fit but don't stick to a regular schedule, or are reasonably fit and do your best to keep moving, one size does not fit all for workout routines. We have asked Matt Natale, an integrative fitness and nutrition practitioner who has a private practice in northern New Jersey, to design three increasingly challenging workouts to suit your level of fitness. Matt was a featured fitness trainer in two episodes of *The Biggest Loser*. But don't worry. We told him that we didn't want killer workouts—we want to get you moving, not cripple you. Matt has dedicated his life to helping and teaching people to feel their very best. He believes that in order to reach your highest potential, you have to commit to cultivating a synergy among mind, body, and spirit. I'll let him introduce the workouts.

> The philosophy of "just move" is smart. Let's, for a moment, compare moving water with stationary water. Moving water is clear, crisp, and inviting, while stationary water is stagnant, cloudy, and smelly. Your body composition is about 60 percent water. Regular movement will keep your body flowing and help bring you optimal health and vibrancy.
>
> Always choose a form of exercise that resonates with you on a physical, emotional, and mental level. Don't force yourself into the latest trendy exercise craze just because everyone else is doing it. Try different exercise programs with an open mind. If you do not connect with a program, just move on to something else—as long as you keep moving.
>
> Set a clear intention before starting an exercise or movement session. Mindless movement will bring you haphazard and scattered results. Take a quiet moment before you start and connect with the reasons you want to be healthy. Crystalize those thoughts and take a deep breath. Your mind and body are now synergized.
>
> Now you are ready.

THE WORKOUTS

Make sure to warm up before performing these exercises. You can warm up for 5 to 10 minutes by dancing, walking, jogging, cycling, rope skipping, playing with the dog, stairclimbing, or anything else that will raise your body temperature.

You can safely perform these exercises three alternate days a week for optimal results.

Beginners Instructions

- Do one exercise at a time, performing 10 repetitions.
- Rest 30 seconds between exercises.
- Rest 1 minute after completing all six of the exercises, which is 1 circuit.
- Do two more circuits, resting 1 minute between circuits.
- Use 3- to 5-pound dumbbells when needed.

EXERCISE 1:
BEGINNERS STANDING
LEG EXTENSIONS

TARGETS: Thighs (quads), hips (hip flexors), core (abdominals), balance

1. Stand on one leg with your arms fully extended to the side.

2. Keep the knee of your supporting leg slightly bent.

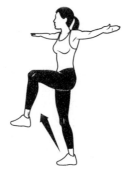

3. Hold your other leg up with a right angle at the hip and knee.

4. Keep your back straight and head level. Keep your chest high and stomach in.

5. Slowly extend your lower leg until you softly lock your knee.

6. Hold for 2 seconds and slowly return your lower leg to the start position.

7. Exhale as you extend your leg and inhale as you return to the start position.

8. Repeat 10 times. Then change legs and repeat 10 times.

EXERCISE 2:
BEGINNERS WALL PUSHUP

TARGETS: Chest (pectorals), back of arms (triceps), shoulders (anterior deltoids)

1. Stand facing a wall with your feet approximately 2 feet away.

2. Position your feet shoulder-width apart.

3. Position your hands a few inches wider than your shoulders on the wall.

4. Keep your back straight and head level.

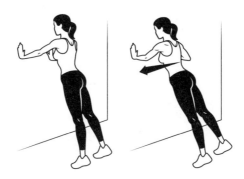

5. Slowly bend your elbows until your nose is about an inch from the wall.

6. Slowly return to a soft lockout at your elbows.

7. Inhale as you come close to the wall and exhale as you push away.

8. Repeat 10 times.

EXERCISE 3:
BEGINNERS PLANK

TARGETS: Core (abdominals), shoulders (erectors and deltoids), back of arms (triceps)

1. Get on your hands and knees.

2. Position your hands directly under your shoulders.

3. Keep your feet together.

4. Keep your back straight, stomach in, and head level.

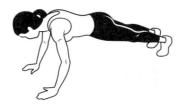

5. Bring your knees off of the ground until only your hands and toes are on the ground.

6. Keep your knees locked and don't hold your breath.

7. Hold for 15 seconds.

8. Repeat 10 times.

EXERCISE 4: BEGINNERS STANDING DUMBBELL CURLS

TARGETS: Front of arms and forearms (biceps)

1. Stand with your feet positioned slightly wider than shoulder width.

2. Keep your knees bent, stomach in, and chest high.

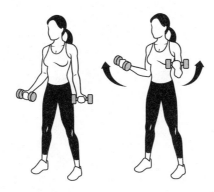

3. Hold the dumbbells at full arm extension with palms facing your sides.

4. Keep your shoulders back and head level.

5. Slowly raise the dumbbells up by bending your elbows. Stop when your elbows are at a right angle.

6. Slowly lower the dumbbells back to a full arm extension.

7. Exhale as you raise the dumbbells up and inhale as you lower them.

8. Repeat 10 times.

EXERCISE 5:
BEGINNERS STANDING
REAR LEG RAISE

TARGETS: Rear end (glutes), lower back (erectors)

1. Stand approximately 24 inches from a wall.

2. Position your feet approximately 12 inches apart.

3. Place your hands against a wall at shoulder height.

4. Keep your head level, stomach in, and chest high.

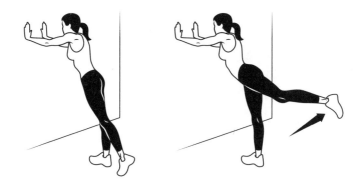

5. Slightly push into the wall as you raise a leg straight behind you.

6. You may bend forward slightly as you raise your leg.

7. Your knee in your supporting leg should be slightly bent.

8. Hold your leg for 2 seconds at the top position.

9. Slowly lower your leg back down to the ground.

10. Exhale as you raise your leg up and inhale as you lower it.

11. Repeat 10 times. Repeat with other leg.

EXERCISE 6:
BEGINNERS STANDING
LATERAL DUMBBELL RAISES

TARGETS: Shoulders (deltoids), upper back (trapezoids)

1. Stand with your feet positioned slightly wider than shoulder width.

2. Keep your knees slightly bent, stomach in, and chest high.

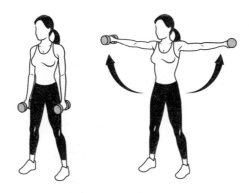

3. Hold the dumbbells at full arm extension at your sides with your palms facing your outer thighs.

4. Keep your shoulders back and head level.

5. Slowly raise the dumbbells out to your sides until the dumbbells are at the level of your shoulders and your palms are facing down.

6. Slowly lower the dumbbells back down to the sides of your thighs.

7. Exhale as you raise the dumbbells and inhale as you lower them.

8. Repeat 10 times.

9. Repeat 2 more circuits of the six Beginners Exercises.

Intermediate Instructions

- Perform 15 repetitions per exercise.
- Go from one exercise to the next with no rest, until you complete all the exercises. That is 1 circuit.
- Rest for 30 seconds and do 3 more full circuits, resting for 30 seconds between each circuit.
- Use 5- to 8-pound dumbbells when needed.

EXERCISE 1:
INTERMEDIATE SQUATS

TARGETS: Thighs (quads), rear end (glutes)

1. Stand with your feet wider than your hips, and your toes pointed slightly outward.

2. Keep your stomach in and chest high. Extend your arms out in front of you, palms down.

3. Keep your head level and back straight.

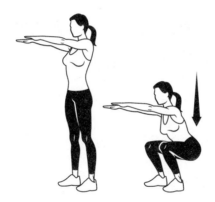

4. Stick your butt backward as you slowly lower yourself.

5. Lean forward slightly as you descend.

6. When your legs are parallel with the floor, stop and return to the top position.

7. Inhale on the way down and exhale on the way up.

8. Repeat 15 times.

EXERCISE 2:
INTERMEDIATE DUMBBELL FLYS

TARGETS: Chest (pectorals), shoulders (deltoids)

1. Position yourself on your back with your knees bent and feet on the floor.

2. Hold the dumbbells above your shoulders with your arms fully extended.

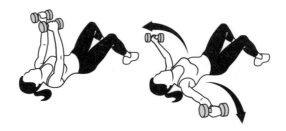

3. Slowly lower the dumbbells out to the sides of your chest.

4. Bend your elbows slightly as your elbows get closer to the floor.

5. When your elbows lightly touch the floor, return to the starting position.

6. Inhale on the way down and exhale as you raise the dumbbells back to the top.

7. Repeat 15 times.

EXERCISE 3:
INTERMEDIATE REVERSE AB CRUNCH

TARGETS: Stomach (abdominals)

1. Position yourself on your back with your hands next to your hips, palms down.

2. Keep your head on the floor.

3. Raise your legs with bent knees in the air.

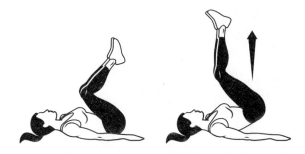

4. Position your bent knees over your lower stomach.

5. Contract your stomach muscles and bring your knees over your chest until your tailbone lifts slightly off of the floor.

6. Do not bend your knees more while you do this.

7. Slowly return to the starting position.

8. Inhale as your knees move over your chest and exhale as you return to the starting position.

9. Repeat 15 times.

EXERCISE 4:
INTERMEDIATE STANDING DUMBBELL OVERHEAD PRESS

TARGETS: Shoulders (deltoids), back of arms (triceps), upper back (trapezoids)

1. Stand with your feet slightly wider than shoulder width.

2. Keep your knees slightly bent, stomach in, and chest high.

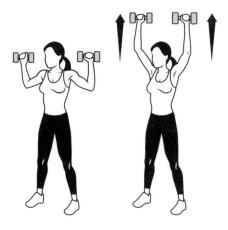

3. Hold the dumbbells at the sides of your shoulders with your palms facing forward and elbows bent.

4. Keep your head level.

5. Slowly push the dumbbells up overhead until your elbows are at a soft lockout.

6. Slowly return the dumbbells to the sides of your shoulders.

7. Exhale as you push the dumbbells up and inhale as you lower them.

8. Repeat 15 times.

EXERCISE 5:
INTERMEDIATE REAR STRAIGHT LEG RAISE

TARGETS: Rear end (glutes), lower back (erectors)

1. Position yourself on your stomach.

2. Rest your turned head on your hands and keep your feet together.

3. Slowly raise a straight leg up into the air as high as you can.

4. Keep your toe pointed and your knee locked.

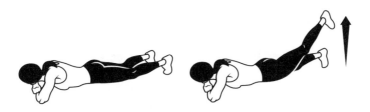

5. Hold the top position for 2 seconds.

6. Slowly return your leg to the ground.

7. Exhale as you raise your leg and inhale as you lower it.

8. Repeat 15 times. Repeat with the other leg.

EXERCISE 6:
INTERMEDIATE BENT-OVER TRICEPS DUMBBELL EXTENSION

TARGETS: Back of arms (triceps), back of shoulders (deltoids)

1. Stand with one foot approximately 3 feet behind the other.

2. The heel of your back foot is off of the floor.

3. Hold a dumbbell in one hand on the same side as your back leg.

4. Lean forward until the forearm of your other arm is resting on top of the thigh of your front leg.

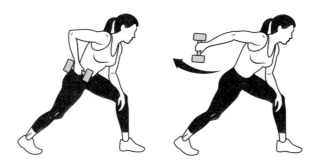

5. Keep your back straight and stomach in.

6. Raise the dumbbell up until your elbow is at a right angle.

7. Now extend your elbow fully to a soft lockout.

8. Slowly return your elbow to a right angle.

9. Exhale as you extend your arm and inhale as you return to the start position.

10. Repeat 15 times. Repeat extension with the other arm.

11. Repeat 2 more circuits of the six Intermediate Exercises.

Advanced Instructions

- Perform 15 repetitions per exercise.
- Hold the plank for 15 seconds each side.
- Do the exercises back to back without rest, until all are completed. That is 1 circuit.
- Perform 4 circuits back to back with no rest.
- Use 10- to 12-pound dumbbells when needed.

EXERCISE 1:
ADVANCED LUNGES

TARGETS: Thighs (quads, hamstrings), hips (hip abductors), rear end (glutes)

1. Position your rear foot about 36 inches behind your front foot.

2. Your rear heel is off of the floor and your front foot is pointed straight ahead.

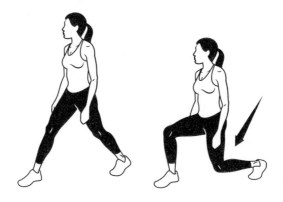

3. Keep both knees slightly bent, stomach in, and chest high.

4. Keep your hands at your sides, shoulders back, and head level.

5. Slowly lower your body straight down until your back knee gets close to the floor.

6. Do not lean forward as you lower yourself.

7. Hold the bottom position for 2 seconds and then slowly return to the top position.

8. Inhale as you lower your body and exhale as you push back up.

9. Repeat 15 times. Switch legs and repeat.

EXERCISE 2:
ADVANCED PUSHUPS

TARGETS: Chest (pectorals), back of arms (triceps), shoulders (deltoids)

1. Lie on your stomach with your feet together.

2. Place your hands several inches wider than your outer chest muscles.

3. Push your body up off of the floor until you softly lock your elbows.

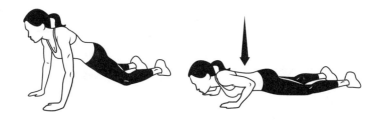

4. Keep your knees on the floor the whole time.

5. If you are strong enough, you can lift your knees off of the floor.

6. Keep your back straight at all times.

7. Slowly lower yourself back to the floor.

8. Take a 1-second break on the floor before the next rep.

9. Exhale on the way up and inhale on the way down.

10. Repeat 15 times.

EXERCISE 3:
ADVANCED PLANK WITH LEG UP

TARGETS: Core (abdominals), rear end (glutes), hips (hip flexors), shoulders (deltoids)

1. Position yourself on your stomach.

2. Fold your hands and fingers together and place them under your face.

3. Position your forearms on the ground and feet together.

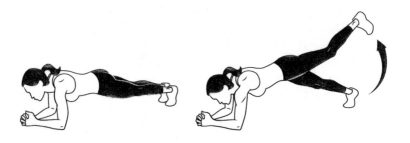

4. Lift your body off of the floor.

5. Keep your back straight and stomach in.

6. While maintaining that position, raise one leg up as high as possible.

7. Keep your foot flexed and knee locked on the raised leg.

8. Hold for 15 seconds and switch legs.

9. Breathe freely.

10. Repeat 15 times.

EXERCISE 4:
ADVANCED BENT-OVER DUMBBELL ROWS

TARGETS: Upper back (lats and traps), lower back (erectors), front of arms (biceps)

1. Stand with your feet approximately 6 inches apart.

2. Hold the dumbbell at your sides with your shoulders back.

3. Hold your stomach in and chest high.

4. Bend over at the waist until your chest is parallel with the floor.

5. Bend your knees several inches.

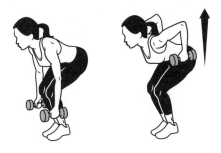

6. Your arms are fully extended, and the dumbbells are lined up under your shoulders.

7. Pull the dumbbells up to the sides of your torso.

8. Slowly lower them back to the start position.

9. Exhale as you raise the dumbbells and inhale as you lower them.

10. Repeat 15 times.

EXERCISE 5:
ADVANCED GLUTE SQUEEZE

TARGETS: Rear end (glutes), back of legs (hamstrings), lower back (erectors)

1. Position yourself on your back with your knees bent and feet on the floor.

2. Your feet are positioned slightly wider than your hips and approximately 12 inches from your butt.

3. Rest your arms at your sides and your head on the floor.

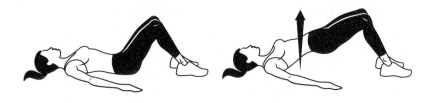

4. Push your entire pelvic region and lower back off of the floor as high as you can.

5. Hold the top position for 2 seconds and squeeze your butt muscles.

6. Slowly lower your pelvic region back to the floor.

7. Exhale as you push up and inhale as you lower yourself.

8. Repeat 15 times.

EXERCISE 6:
ADVANCED TRICEPS DIPS

TARGETS: Back of arms (triceps), shoulders (deltoids), chest (pectorals)

1. Sit on the edge of a stable chair.

2. Position your hands on the sides of the chair.

3. Move your body away from the chair, supporting your weight with your straight arms.

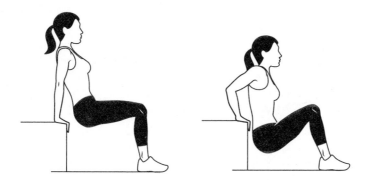

4. Your knees are at a right angle and your feet are flat on the floor.

5. Slowly lower yourself by bending at the elbow.

6. As you lower yourself, keep your back close to the chair.

7. Keep your chest high, stomach in, and head level.

8. When your elbows reach a right angle, return to the top position.

9. Inhale as you lower yourself and exhale as you push up.

10. Repeat 15 times.

11. Repeat 3 more circuits of the 6 Advanced Exercises.

Just like everything else, keep it slow and steady. Consistency counts a lot. You will see changes in the way you move if you keep it up. You want to be supple and strong so that you can move through the world with energy and grace. Gravity will take its toll on your body if you don't fight it. Keep moving to stay healthy.

To feel your best, you have to exercise every aspect of yourself—your mind and spirit need a workout as much as your body does. To live your life to the fullest, you have to break out of conventional thinking about what aging is, because it's what you want it to be. You have a choice.

There is a fountain of youth: it is your mind, your talents, the creativity you bring to your life and the lives of people you love. When you learn to tap this source, you will truly have defeated age. —Sophia Loren

We have negative mental habits that come up over and over again. One of the most significant negative habits we should be aware of is that of constantly allowing our mind to run off into the future. . . . We may have fears about the future because we don't know how it's going to turn out, and these worries and anxieties keep us from enjoying being here now. —Thich Nhat Hanh

CHAPTER

12

Living Life to the Fullest

It's time for an attitude adjustment. You can view this period as the beginning of the end or you can look at the rest of your life as a gift. You can choose to be engaged and vital rather than resigned and on the sidelines. Your life can be what you want to make it. You know what's not working for you. You trust yourself enough to figure out what you really want, and you are savvy enough to go for it. This, at last, is the payoff for a lifetime of hard work—now you can live your dreams. You don't have to define yourself by what you've done. Now that you know what really matters, you can reinvent your life. You can find new passions, keep learning, expand your circle of friends, and spend some of your free time helping others.

The last part of your life is a time to be adventurous. What are you afraid of? Don't let your fears narrow your experience. Take a chance. Make a list of things you have always wanted to do and work your way through it. Whether it's learning more about modern art or trekking the Himalayas, nothing is holding you back. What is wonderful about this time of life is that you can continue to learn. Study a new language, learn to tango, adopt a rescue dog, improve your computer skills, make a garden. There is so much to do if you think about it.

As you probably have noticed by now, I'm not the type who will spend the rest of my life stuck in "I woulda, coulda, shoulda" thinking. Though I have my moments of anger, fear, and frustration, I don't let regret linger in my life for long. I look forward, not back. Success is the greatest revenge. I don't waste time and energy. When bad things happen, I don't let it consume me. I'd rather focus on making things better. I refuse to let negativity take me over. I don't want the kindness taken out of me.

I know many women who have become bitter and angry when their husbands leave them for a younger woman. They believe their lives are over and stop growing completely. They become so negative that it's hard to be around them. What do children learn about life when they see their mothers in this mental and emotional state? Abandonment is emotionally crippling—I don't want to make light of what these women are going through. Their sense of loss is devastating. But being miserable is not hurting anyone but themselves. Then there are the former beauty queens who are now 30 pounds overweight and would rather live with the memory of how they used to be than do something right now to be their best.

You get to choose the way you live during your third act. It's all about attitude and what you make of any situation. I figure I have one-third of my life left, and I'm not going to waste a minute of it. When things don't work out the way I want, I pick myself up and am on to the next thing. It's painful, but I've learned to get over disappointments and failures with a minimum of drama.

The story of my wine business, which I mentioned at the beginning of the book, is a good example. I was approached to start a wine company several years ago. When I listened to the pitch, I had an immediate and strong reaction. It was like winning a pinball game—the lights were flashing and the bells were ringing. From my days in France, I knew a lot about good eating and drinking—especially wine and cheese. This felt so right. After all, 26 years earlier, I named my first-born Margaux after Chateau Margaux and bought two cases of that exceptional wine in 1979, a very good year. I had been offered a great adventure!

I'd never tried going into any other business besides acting. Many companies had approached me about endorsing makeup, hair products, and jewelry, but nothing ever hit me. Being named the ugliest girl on the bus in the sixth grade had stayed with me. I felt I'd be a fraud selling beauty products. But selling wine was something else, and the timing was right. When the business would be ready to launch, *The Sopranos* would be winding down and the kids would be mostly out of the house. It was a perfect fit. I knew this was a business I could throw myself into heart and soul.

I told my future partners that I couldn't sell wines I didn't like. To begin, I had to go to Italy to select the wines. I either liked a wine or I didn't. I wasn't going to base my choices on production costs or price range. I would go with what I loved, and I would have final say. They agreed, and I went for it.

I knew I couldn't do this alone, so I approached my brother, who had retired young from his job as a VP of a medical instruments company, and asked him to help. He said, "No, you don't go into business with family. It's a bad idea."

"You're going to do this," I insisted.

His answer remained, "No."

"Don't make me call Mommy and Daddy," I threatened. "You retired at 58. You don't even play golf. What are you going to do with your time?"

Sal finally broke down and agreed to help me. I enlisted Monica to join the team. We took a 10-day trip with our new partners to visit vineyards in different regions of Italy. It was a wonderful trip. We went through Tuscany, Piedmont, Puglia, and many other regions in Italy. I selected eight or nine different wines at a range of prices. We had a Montepulciano, a Barolo, a Brunello di Montalcino, an old vines Primitivo, a Pinot Grigio, an Amarone, and a Chianti Classico Reserve. Our distributor was going to sell the wines in New Jersey, New York, Pennsylvania, Florida, Nevada, and Illinois.

We made our scouting trip to Italy in 2005. Martha Stewart sent filming equipment with us for material to air on her show and had me on several times to talk about wine. We launched Bracco Wines in June 2006 with an appearance on the first season of *Top Chef.* I was also on the season finale with the wines. We didn't have a marketing budget—I called in favors from friends and family. Mayor Bloomberg came to our New York opening. The Hard Rock Café in Florida and New York City threw several parties to feature our wines. I was interviewed for *Wine Spectator* and appeared on *Conan* and *The View* to talk about Bracco Wines.

Based in a small office I rented in New York, we traveled all over the country working like dogs to sell Bracco Wines. I'm talking about 5 days a week on the road for months. Restaurant and casino owners, who featured our wines on their wine lists, served us huge meals. Everyone wanted to feed me. We treated buyers to lavish dinners and wine tastings. I can't tell you how many appearances I made at liquor stores and supermarkets like Publix in Florida to promote the wines. To my surprise, people lined up and asked me to sign their bottles. Countless meals to court buyers, jet lag, room service, and mini-bars took their toll. My weight started to climb.

Along the way, I met the famous Mel Dick, the almost 80-year-old president of the wine division of Southern Wine and Spirits, and his wonderful wife, Bobbi. After Robert Parker, he is the most powerful person in the wine industry. To work out, he boxed with Angelo Dundee, who trained Muhammad Ali and Sugar Ray Leonard. I was so impressed. He was a boy from Brooklyn who had a vision. It was love at first sight for me—those sparkling blue eyes got me. He is a man who is passionate about what he does, and that keeps him young. He lives life with real gusto. He's a gatherer of fascinating people of all ages and surrounds himself with them. Being with him is always a lot of fun. I always gravitate to older people like that, because that's how I want to be.

I was getting an MBA in the wine business—selling, merchandising, and marketing—from on-the-ground experience but couldn't get the numbers or find out what was going on. One day, Sal sat me down and told me there was no question in his mind that we needed an exit strategy.

I was so hurt and disappointed. I had dragged my brother and Monica along for the ride. We had put our blood, sweat, and tears into this business for 3 years. I just ached. I knew the wine company would have worked, but I had to face the fact that I would never know my full potential in business. This was a real kick in the ass. I was so upset with myself.

Just as the business came tumbling down, my parents' chronic physical problems got serious. I was working so hard that my relationship with my boyfriend fell apart. I was also running back and forth to Los Angeles for my role on *Rizzoli & Isles*. During those 3 years, my much-loved house in Snedens Landing was on the market. My mother always said that the minute I sold the house, they would leave me. The house sold in the winter of 2012, and they died shortly after.

Losing them within 9 days of each other, I was bereft. I had no one to go home to. I never felt more alone. I had no boyfriend, no husband, no parents, and my children were grown. It was a perfect storm—physically, emotionally, and mentally. It was one of the roughest moments of my life. But then I looked at my daughters and realized I had reasons beyond my own fears to stay healthy. That revved up my fighting spirit. I could not give up. I wanted to be healthy and fit into all my old clothes. You know the story from here. My friend Lisa recommended jump-starting the changes I wanted to make with a liver cleanse. The rest is history.

My transformation experience was so powerful, I still want to stop people on the street and recommend that they try the Clean Up Your Act Plan. Helping women and men who want to stay healthy as they age has become my new mission. People need support and encouragement to live life to the fullest.

After my weight gain, several weight loss companies offered me a bundle of money to become a spokesperson for their programs. When I studied their products, I was surprised by the number of chemicals on the ingredient lists. How were these foods supposed to make me healthy? I wanted to do a lot more for myself than just lose weight. Improving my health and preventing future problems were my real goals. I didn't think I'd get there by consuming chemical cocktails. I turned down the offers. I couldn't back a product that I didn't believe in.

Before I did the liver cleanse Lisa suggested, I studied the product labels. I was impressed by how clean the protein shake, vitamins and minerals, and phytonutrients she gave me were. The ingredients were all vegetable based. **I knew I needed the best to become the best I could be.** As you have read in the Real Time Change comments from the women who tried the plan for 6 weeks, this program works. Those women were able to recapture the lightness, pride, clarity, and joy that they thought they had lost for good. I created my Liv4Mor brand with Lisa so that more people could benefit from such a powerfully nutritious cleanse.

Even after my experience with the wine company, I'm not gun-shy about committing myself to a new enterprise. I'm not holding back—I want to use everything I can to get my healing message out. I am going public with the news that it's never too late to improve how you look, feel, and live. **Helping women and men to stay vital and energetic has become my passion and the focus of my third act. I never would have predicted the direction my life has taken. That's the point. You never know where you are headed or what is in store for you tomorrow. You just never know what's coming. It doesn't have to be a disaster. If you stay open, you can find new meaning and fill your life with new interests.**

I have to laugh. My daughter Stella is so much like me. I'm actually Stella-Big. College wasn't working for her, so she dropped out. She was never interested in school. I said, "Fine, but you're not having a 4-year vacation on my dollar. Get a job." She has worked for 5 years at Intermix, a terrific clothing store. She has a talent for putting together stylish looks for older customers helping them to see themselves differently and to take some chances. Of course, she's had a lot of experience from dressing her mother! She attracted a long list of regular customers who appreciated her sensitivity, dedication, and great sense of style. She eventually learned that supporting yourself in the real world is not so easy, and being back in school looked good. She understood the value of education and the confidence and feeling of self-worth that education brings. She wanted to confirm she could do it. It was unfinished business for her that she wanted to complete.

She had to start over from scratch. She was the oldest person in all her classes. She did very well and got her degree, and decided to go on for graduate work in clinical psychology. She was accepted in a very competitive program. At 28, she expects to be the oldest one in her grad school class. But that's not stopping her. She's on a mission just like me. Stella believes that everyone should be educated. She volunteers for a program at a women's prison and teaches inmates math. It means a lot to her to help others get an education.

Stella, Margaux, and I share the same determination. Margaux graduated from New York University and worked in business for a few years before deciding to go back for an MBA, which she did at Wharton. Not only is she a new mother, but she started a company that is developing wearable technology for women. I'm so proud of both my girls.

The lesson is to believe that you deserve better whatever your age. You really have to want it and be willing to do whatever you can to get it. Everyone has disappointments and failures in life, but you can't let them stop you. You have to confront how you are feeling directly. **Say to yourself, "I don't want to be like this—I want to be like that," as you point to the stars. You have to keep reaching if you want to stay vibrant and powerful. Remember, the challenge and the struggle are what make life interesting.** You have to want to be present and know in your gut that you are worthwhile.

LESS IS MORE

Some people measure getting older as a losing proposition. I believe that your third act is a time of change, not a series of reductions. **This period of your life is not a gap or a lack but an opportunity. Things will be different, but you don't have to resign yourself to less of anything.** Your third act has little to do with being in the game. It's a new chapter, which you can write however you want to. Aging gracefully is liberating. You're the boss of your time and creativity, and you have earned it.

If your children have left the nest, do you really need the stress of keeping up the house in which you brought up your kids? Sure, there are millions of memories, but it's okay to let the place go. Get rid of that clutter—clear the decks. What you have does not define you at a certain point. Keep it simple, sister.

After our parents' deaths, my brother, sister, and I went through the house. It was amazing to see how much they had held on to. We each kept a few pieces and keepsakes, but we gave most of the contents of their house to people who needed the things and what was left to the Salvation Army. **It became clear to me that having all that stuff weighs you down financially and emotionally. That's why I have downsized in Los Angeles. I want my life to be easier and simpler—cozy with a view beats grand. Having less is a positive for me.**

Facing retirement seems like the same kind of loss to people. Ageism is alive and well in the marketplace, especially in tough financial times. Many of us will be working longer than our parents did. Retirement might not be an option for financial reasons. Some people are passionate about what they do and never plan to stop working. It's unquestionably harder to work when you are older. Thank God that Hollywood is not a microcosm, or most of the country over 35 would be unemployed.

If you have been married to your job and are used to being fueled by stress, you can learn to enjoy the luxury of more free time in your third act. Many of us working women have been juggling the demands of work and home, but once the children leave the nest, a lot of time opens up. You might have to learn to enjoy it! Baby boomers have been so driven to be successful. It's such a relief to look forward to having the time to relax and just look out the window if you want to and not to be constantly striving to achieve.

Explore—the world is wide open to you, and there are so many possibilities you have probably never considered. It's not, "Sixty—I'm done." Push yourself. You can occupy your mind, body, and spirit with things you love to do. Who told you there is an age limit to creativity? **There isn't a set point at which you become the best you will ever be. Your criteria evolve and change with the passage of time. When I received the first envelope from AARP, I threw it out.** *They made a mistake,* **I thought.** *It can't be for me.* **Now, I'm interested!**

There is no reason the last third of your life should not be more than the first two-thirds. I always want to sit with exciting older people at dinner. They have so much to offer. One of my favorite dashing men is 95 years old. Alive and kicking, he still does business deals. He does not stop. Full of stories and ideas, he is always fascinating to be around. My parents were the same way. Before they got sick, my friends were crazy about them and enjoyed spending time with them. They were always interested and interesting. I want to be that kind of person when I am old. Keep those cute guys around me and coming back for more!

My brother did something I admire after he retired. He went to school to become an EMT (emergency medical technician). He was worried that he wasn't strong enough to carry or lift patients and asked me how to build up his strength. I suggested Pilates and swimming, which work everything. He applied himself and now serves his community with confidence. Who says the world stops when you retire? **You can do just about anything you want as long as you stay healthy. If you don't have your health, you will lose your stamina and your zest for life. The trade-off seems like a no-brainer to me. You have to focus** on prevention and the health you can control. **Eat well and keep moving to live well!**

GIVING BACK IS MORE THAN JUST WRITING A CHECK

If you find yourself with time to fill, don't sit at home watching TV. Charitable organizations are on their knees begging people to help. It doesn't have to mean big contributions. You can donate time. Think of how much you can do to help the vets from the Vietnam and Middle Eastern wars. These soldiers risked their lives and suffered injuries to protect us, and our society is treating them very badly. We have really let them down. My brother wanted to give blood every month at a VA hospital near him, but could not because of a medication he takes. Instead, he volunteers at the same hospital doing menial things people need to have done, and some of those things are not very pretty. But when he thinks about what these people have sacrificed for their country, he wishes he could do more to help.

When our parents were in rehab centers, we knew everybody and would stop in to visit and hold someone's hand for a while. Dominic Chianese, who was in *The Godfather* and played Uncle Junior on *The Sopranos*, started to show up at nursing homes and assisted living centers with his guitar and sang for the elderly. He sang at my parents' funerals. What a beautiful voice he has! The old people enjoyed the entertainment so much that he started an organization called Joy through Art 40 years ago to provide entertainment at senior facilities. He hires fellow singers, unemployed actors who would otherwise be delivering pizza, to go into homes and do sing-alongs. Dominic is treating the elderly with love and respect and bringing them a lot of joy. That is a tremendous gift.

You can volunteer to deliver Meals on Wheels to the homebound, people who often sit alone all day. I knew a man who delivered Meals on Wheels until his death at 89. To the end, he wanted to help others, and it kept him young. There are so many things you can do to help: read to the elderly or sick in homes, rehab centers, hospitals, or hospices or be part of a pet visit team. **Let's not abandon our old people. They deserve our attention.**

The wisdom you have gained living life puts you in a unique position. You have so much to pass on to others. Think of all the abused and underprivileged kids, especially teenagers, who could benefit from what you know. Exposing them to new ideas and the good things in life will give them a better chance. You can volunteer at tutoring programs or as grandparents in the classroom. You can be a big brother or sister and take kids to sports events, museums, movies, and other cultural events. There are so many children in need. I'm on the board for The Felix Organization/Adoptees for Children, which provides opportunities and experiences for kids growing up in the foster care system. Those kids get lost so easily. You can mentor people starting out in your field. **You are never too old to share your life experience with young people. And you could learn a thing or two from them!**

I was on the board of directors of Robert Kennedy Jr.'s environmental organization, Riverkeeper. Working to clean up the environment is so important, and that can be as simple as picking up trash and dog poop on the street. You can become more politically active locally and work for your party during elections. You can raise money for your favorite charity. I'm involved with the Rockland County Women's Shelter that helps abused women. I try to help anyone who looks needy. We ended up taking a lower offer for my parents' house because the family had a young child and one on the way. We decided to give them a chance in life with their first house. We know our parents would have wanted to give these people their home.

No matter how you direct your energy to helping others, you will receive so much more than you give. You have the chance to make the world a better place and to leave a lasting legacy. I'd call that lucky. If you can say, "I am still a vibrant, contributing human being, and I am not dead yet," that's saying a lot. Those words are my mantra and my hope for the years ahead.

All of us were brought up with this view of life like an arc. You're born, you peak at midlife, then you decline into decrepitude. It's a downward slope. You're "over the hill." And I realized, yeah, I'm over the hill, but look at all these other hills—no one told me there were gonna be all these hills! And I can climb them!
—Jane Fonda

I never lose sight of the fact that just being is fun.
—Katharine Hepburn

AFTERWORD

Run with It

I hope you are fired up to reclaim yourself and stay full of life for the long haul. As you take one slow and steady step at a time on the path to renewed health, energy, and contentment, have faith in your body's miraculous ability to heal itself. You just have to stop overloading its systems with toxins, sugar, and stress to allow your body to function as it was meant to. You have to get off your butt and use those muscles before they go slack. Mental activity counts, too. To stay sharp, you want to keep those brain neurons firing, so challenge your mind by exposing yourself to new things and by staying in touch with what is happening in the world. Always make sure to have friends much older and much younger than yourself, as I do. I'm inspired and stimulated by the young and the elderly people in my life. There is nothing like a different point of view to give you perspective. I know I learn a lot from people at both ends of the age timeline.

A positive, curious mind will find wonder and beauty everywhere, even in the simplest things. When you lose your sense of wonder, you lose your joy. It really is time to stop and smell the roses. If you don't now, you will miss so much. Appreciating the everyday things you take for granted will keep your spirits high. Be present in the moment with every ounce of your being. Feel the sun on your skin, enjoy quenching your thirst with a glass of cold water, make preparing dinner a sensual experience—for me, taking in the colors, textures, and aromas is as satisfying as the meal itself. You want to spend the time you have left living life to the fullest.

We have laid down the rejuvenation plan that saved me, in the simplest way possible. When you follow the 14-day cleanse, you will see and feel remarkable results that will make you want to eat clean forever. We gave you a road map for eating clean for the rest of your life with the Clean Up Your Act Diet. We went beyond the "how-tos" and provided you with the "whys," because knowing what is hurting you will give you the determination to change. Breaking habits is never easy, but being able to fast-forward and see that the aches and pains of today can develop into chronic illness and accelerated aging is a big motivator. Understanding why you are dropping sugar, dairy, GMOs, caffeine, gluten, and white foods from your diet makes what you are doing seem a gift to yourself, not a sacrifice.

We have done our best to include in one book all you need to know to slow the aging process and restore your glow. We've distilled a tremendous amount of information in these pages. We wanted you to have a reference you can keep on a bookshelf or next to your bed to refer to often.

I was elated to witness the success of the 14 women who volunteered to try the program. Though Lisa has worked with thousands of people and has turned lives around, I only had my experience to go on. Rodale set up a Facebook page so that we could talk to each other during the 6 weeks. It was great fun! We were able to connect, support each other, and share tips. Having a community is easier than going it alone. I'm so eager to hear what the Clean Up Your Act Plan does for you. You have to let me know how it goes. We've set up our Web site, tothefullestbook.com, so that you can tell us about the ups and downs of your experience. You can also communicate with others who are doing, or have done, the cleanse and have converted to eating clean. We'll keep a stream of information, recipes, and inspiration going to help you stick to your guns. You'll also be able to order Liv4Mor products from the Web site and find out where the products are available.

You made one of the best decisions of your life when you chose to clean up your act. Don't expect to be perfect. Just keep the goal in mind and make corrections whenever you have to. Your healthy way of life will show in how you look and feel. You will become a force of nature—powerful and in control of your destiny. I want you to be fully alive and to appreciate every minute of it. That's a life worth living!

ACKNOWLEDGMENTS

So many people, working together, helped to make this book a reality. I couldn't have had a better team.

My book wouldn't be what it is without the remarkable women who followed the program for 6 weeks. Their experiences made me even more confident about the program. They were sophisticated, funny, and really sharp. Diane Arpino, Stephanie Augello, Elizabeth Bloom, Michele Bloom, Helyn L. Bryant, Lucille Ircha, Amy Murphy, Dale Lawrence, Iliana Guibert McGinnis, Ana Napoles, Wendy Napoles, Jeanie Ciuppa Santacroce, Loretta Lang Stokes, and Mary Lampe Suddell—I am grateful to all of you for taking a leap and trying the program. Your insights and comments brought tears to my eyes. You are great women! I am glad the Clean Up Your Act Plan made a big difference in your lives—without exception. And thanks to Michele Stanten, who made it all happen.

Lisa, Heather, and Monica, without the three of you—your love, compassion, and years of guidance—I wouldn't have had this great life.

Thanks to David Vigliano, my literary agent, who introduced me to Diane Reverand. She captured my voice and my passion and was a "Jill-of-all-trades." I know she worked hard writing this book, but more important, she made me go to the hospital when the swelling from a bee sting was slowly creeping up my arm. I'd do anything to avoid a tetanus shot, but she didn't let me get away with it.

Thank you, Fred Pescatore, for thinking, feeling, and living what I describe in the book.

Thanks to everyone at Rodale. Jennifer Levesque, my editor, has been enthusiastic from the start—and a good boxing partner. Her assistant, Christopher DeMarchis, is a paragon of thoughtfulness and efficiency. Mary Ann Naples, publisher, and Kristin Kiser, deputy publisher, encouraged us every step of the way. Amy King not only worked on the design but also participated in the trial group with her husband, Trace Murphy, the only guy brave enough to do it. I also want to acknowledge the Rodale PR/marketing team, including Brent Gallenberger, Melissa Olund, Aly Mostel, Emily Weber Eagan, and Susan Turner as well as my publicist, Claire Mercuri, who are dedicated to getting the word out.

I appreciate the contributions of Matt Natale, Josh McKible, Mark Schafer, and Kathryn Macleod.

Margaux, Stella, Deric, Baby Viv, take a bow. Without you, I would be nothing.

SELECTED SOURCES

Chapter 3 The Hunger Within

Hatfield, Heather. "Emotional Eating: Feeding Your Feelings." WebMD. Reviewed on November 11, 2003. prohealth.com/library/showarticle.cfm?libid=6156.

Helpguide.org. "Emotional Eating: How to Recognize and Stop Emotional Eating." Last updated June 2014. helpguide.org/life/emotional_eating_stress_cravings.htm.

Kotz, Deborah. "Stop Emotional Eating with These 5 Tips." *US News & World Report*, September 22, 2011. http://Health.usnews.com/health-news/diet-fitness/diet/slideshows/stop-emotional-eating-with-these-5-tips/.

Kromberg, Jennifer. "Emotional Eating? 5 Reasons You Can't Stop." *Inside Out* (blog), *Psychology Today*, September 18, 2013. psychologytoday.com/blog/inside-out/201309/emotional-eating-5-reasons-you-can-t-stop.

Lu, Henry C. *Traditional Chinese Medicine: An Authoritative and Comprehensive Guide*. Laguna Beach, CA: Basic Health Publications, 2005.

Maciocia, Giovanni. *The Psyche in Chinese Medicine: Treatment of Emotional and Mental Disharmonies with Acupuncture and Chinese Herbs*. London: Churchill Livingstone, 2009.

Chapter 4 Navigating the Food Maze

DeLuz, Roni, and James Hester, with Diane Reverand. *1 Pound a Day: The Martha's Vineyard Diet Detox and Plan for a Lifetime of Healthy Eating*. New York: Gallery Books, 2013.

Fuhrman, Joel. *Eat to Live: The Amazing Nutrient-Rich Program for Fast and Sustained Weight Loss*. Rev. ed. New York: Little, Brown and Company, 2011.

Hyman, Mark. *Ultra-Metabolism: The Simple Plan for Automatic Weight Loss*. New York: Atria Books, 2008.

Hyman, Mark, and Mark Liponis. *Ultra-Prevention: The 6-Week Plan That Will Make You Healthy for Life*. New York: Atria Books, 2005.

Kessler, David A. *The End of Overeating: Taking Control of the Insatiable American Appetite*. New York: Rodale, 2009.

Nestle, Marion. *Food Politics: How the Food Industry Influences Nutrition and Health*. Rev. ed. Berkeley: University of California Press, 2007.

Pollan, Michael. *In Defense of Food: An Eater's Manifesto*. New York: Penguin Books, 2009.

Pollan, Michael. *The Omnivore's Dilemma: A Natural History of Four Meals*. New York: Penguin Books, 2007.

Processed Foods

Denny, Sharon. "Avoiding Processed Foods? Surprise! This Is Processed, Too!" Academy of Nutrition and Dietetics. Reviewed on May 2014. eatright.org/Public/content.aspx?id=6442471055.

"50 Other Names for Sugar." Organic Authority, April 3, 2013. organicauthority.com/health/50-other-names-for-sugar.html.

Freudenberg, Nicholas. *Lethal but Legal: Corporations, Consumption, and Protecting Public Health.* New York: Oxford University Press, 2014.

Goodwin, Jeremy. "257 Names for Hidden Sugar." My Fitness Pal. myfitnesspal.com/topics/show/821596-257-names-for-hidden-sugar.

Gunnars, Kris. "9 Ways That Processed Foods Are Slowly Killing People." Authority Nutrition, January 15, 2014. http://authoritynutrition.com/9-ways-that-processed-foods-are-killing-people.

Harvard School of Public Health Nutrition Source. "Added Sugar in the Diet." hsph.harvard.edu/nutritionsource/carbohydrates/added-sugar-in-the-diet/.

Lima, Cristiano. "The 57 Names of Sugar." *Prevention.* prevention.com/food/healthy-eating-tips/57-names-sugar.

Lustig, Robert H. *Fat Chance: Beating the Odds Against Sugar, Processed Food, Obesity, and Disease.* New York: Hudson Street Press, 2013.

Moss, Michael. *Salt, Sugar, Fat: How the Food Giants Hooked Us.* New York: Random House, 2013.

GMOs

Black, Jane. "Foods as Nature Made Them." *Prevention,* March 2012. prevention.com/food/smart-shopping/genetically-modified-foods-what-you-need-know.

Ettinger, Jill. "Are Genetically Modified Foods Causing a Rise in Food Allergies? Organic Authority, January 8, 2012. organicauthority.com/health/are-genetically-modified-foods-gmos-causing-rise-food-allergies.html.

Ettinger, Jill. "Everything You Absolutely Need to Know about GMOS." Organic Authority, February 20, 2012. organicauthority.com/foodie-buzz/what-are-gmos-genetically-modified-crops-foods.html.

Green America. "9 GMO Ingredients to Avoid." http://action.greenamerica.org/p/salsa/web/common/public/signup?signup_page_KEY=7608&tag=adwords&gclid=CMu13dyr7sACFUNgMgodV0sADQ.

Institute for Responsible Technology. "10 Reasons to Avoid GMOs." responsibletechnology.org/10-Reasons-to-Avoid-GMOs.

Krimsky, Sheldon, ed., and Jeremy Gruber, ed. *The GMO Deception: What You Need to Know about the Food, Corporations, and Government Agencies Putting Our Families and Our Environment at Risk.* New York: Skyhorse Publishing, 2014.

Non-GMO Project. "GMO Facts: Frequently Asked Questions." nongmoproject.org/learn-more/.

Smith, Jeffrey M. *Genetic Roulette: The Documented Health Risks of Genetically Engineered Foods.* Fairfield, IA: Yes! Books, 2007.

Smith, Jeffrey. "Genetically Engineered Foods May Cause Rising Food Allergies—Genetically Engineered Soybeans." Institute for Responsible Technology, May 2007. responsibletechnology.org/gmo-dangers/health-risks/articles-about-risks-by-jeffrey-smith/Genetically-Engineered-Foods-May-Cause-Rising-Food-Allergies-Genetically-Engineered-Soybeans-May-2007.

Smith, Jeffrey M. *Seeds of Deception: Exposing Industry and Government Lies about the Safety of the Genetically Engineered Foods You're Eating.* Fairfield, IA: Yes! Books, 2003.

Zerbe, Leah. "7 Things You Need to Know about GMOs." *Prevention*, April 2013. prevention.com/print/33726.

Organic vs. Conventional

American Cancer Society. "Recombinant Bovine Growth Hormone." cancer.org/cancer/cancercauses/othercarcinogens/athome/recombinant-bovine-growth-hormone.

"Animals Raised Organically Are Not Given Growth Hormones or Antibiotics." Natural Society. http://naturalsociety.com/animals-raised-organically-are-not-given-growth-hormones-or-antibiotics/

"Choosing Organic: The Commotion about Organic vs. Conventional Foods." *A Healthier Hokie: A Blog for Smarter Eating* (blog). http://vtnutrition.wordpress.com/facts/organic-vs-conventional-foods/.

Hoffman, Matthew. "Safer Food for a Healthier You." WebMD (in collaboration with Healthy Child Healthy World). Reviewed on December 18, 2008. webmd.com/diet/features/safer-food-healthier-you.

"How to Substitute Sugar." *My Real Food Life (blog)*, December 9, 2011. myrealfoodlife.com/part-3-how-to-substitute-sugar.

Mayo Clinic Staff. "Nutrition and Healthy Eating: Discover the Real Difference between Organic Foods and Their Traditionally Grown Counterparts When It Comes to Nutrition, Safety and Price." Mayo Clinic, June 9, 2014. mayoclinic.org/healthy-living/nutrition-and-healthy-eating/in-depth/organic-food/art-20043880?p=1.

"Meat Eater's Guide to Climate Change+Health: Frequently Asked Questions." Environmental Work Group. ewg.org/meateatersguide/frequently-asked-questions/.

O'Brien, Robyn. "What Corn-Eating Cows Are Doing to Our Health." *Inspired Bites* (blog), *Prevention*, July 10, 2012. http://blogs.prevention.com/inspired-bites/2012/07/10/corned-beef-what-corn-eating-cows-are-doing-to-our-health/.

Organic Consumers Association. "Why We Should All Eat More Organic Food." https://organicconsumers.org/newsletter/organic-bytes-206-2010-year-eating-organically/why-we-should-all-eat-more-organic-food.

"Organic FAQs." *Nature* 428 (April 22, 2004): 796–98. nature.com/nature/journal/v428/n6985/full/428796a.html.

Parnes, Robin Brett. "How Organic Food Works." HowStuffWorks. http://science.howstuffworks.com/environmental/green-science/organic-food7.htm/printable.

Raloff, Janet. "Hormones: Here's the Beef: Environmental Concerns Reemerge over Steroids Given to Livestock." *Science News* 161, no. 1 (January 5, 2002): 10. phschool.com/science/science_news/articles/hormones_beef.html.

Singer, Peter, and Jim Mason. *The Ethics of What We Eat: Why Our Food Choices Matter.* New York: Rodale Books, 2007.

Storrs, Carina. "Hormones In Food: Should You Worry?" Health.com, January 31, 2011. huffingtonpost.com/2011/01/31/hormones-in-food-should-y_n_815385.html.

"Superbugs Invade American Supermarkets." Environmental Work Group, April 2013. ewg.org/meateatersguide/superbugs.

Gluten

American Diabetes Association. "What Foods Have Gluten?" diabetes.org/food-and-fitness/food/planning-meals/gluten-free-diets/what-foods-have-gluten.html.

Davis, William. *Wheat Belly: Lose the Wheat, Lose the Weight, and Find Your Path Back to Health.* New York: Rodale Books, 2011.

FDA. "Gluten-Free Now Means What It Says." August 5, 2014. fda.gov/forconsumers/consumerupdates/ucm363069.htm.

GlutenFree.com Editorial Staff. "What Does Gluten-Free Mean?" August 2013. glutenfree.com/#/articles/what-does-gluten-free-mean.

Mayo Clinic Staff. "Gluten-Free Diet: What's Allowed, What's Not." mayoclinic.org/healthy-living/nutrition-and-healthy-eating/in-depth/gluten-free-diet/art-20048530.

Perlmutter, David, and Kristin Loberg. *Grain Brain: The Surprising Truth about Wheat, Carbs, and Sugar—Your Brain's Silent Killers.* New York: Little, Brown and Company, 2013.

Sanfilippo, Diane. *Practical Paleo: A Customized Approach to Health and a Whole-Foods Lifestyle.* Las Vegas: Victory Belt Publishing, 2012.

Sugar

Alexander, Anne. *The Sugar Smart Diet: Stop Cravings and Lose Weight While Still Enjoying the Sweets You Love!* New York: Rodale, 2013.

American Heart Association. "Sugar-Sweetened Drinks Associated with Higher Blood Pressure." ScienceDaily, March 1, 2011. sciencedaily.com/releases/2011/02/110228163030.htm.

Chen, L. et al. "Reducing Consumption of Sugar-Sweetened Beverages Is Associated with Reduced Blood Pressure: A Prospective Study Among United States Adults." *Circulation* 121 (2010): 2398–2406. http://circ.ahajournals.org/content/121/22/2398.full.

Corliss, Julie. "Eating Too Much Added Sugar Increases the Risk of Dying with Heart Disease." *Harvard Health Blog*, February 6, 2014. health.harvard.edu/blog/eating-too-much-added-sugar-increases-the-risk-of-dying-with-heart-disease-201402067.

Dana-Farber Cancer Institute. "Sugar and Cancer Cells: Ask the Nutritionist." dana-farber.org/Health-Library/Sugar-and-Cancer-Cells.aspx.

Dufty, William. *Sugar Blues.* New York: Grand Central, 1986.

Gardner, Amanda. "Sugar, Not Just Salt, Linked to High Blood Pressure." Health.com, July 1, 2010. cnn.com/2010/HEALTH/07/01/glucose.blood.pressure/.

Gunnars, Kris. "10 Disturbing Reasons Why Sugar Is Bad for You." Authority Nutrition. http://authoritynutrition.com/10-disturbing-reasons-why-sugar-is-bad.

Howard, Barbara, and Judith Wylie-Rosett. "Sugar and Cardiovascular Disease: A Statement for Healthcare Professionals from the Committee on Nutrition of the Council on Nutrition, Physical Activity, and Metabolism of the American Heart Association." *Circulation* 106 (2002): 523–7. http://circ.ahajournals.org/content/106/4/523.full.

Hyman, Mark. *The Blood Sugar Solution 10-Day Detox Diet: Activate Your Body's Natural Ability to Burn Fat and Lose Weight Fast.* New York: Little, Brown and Company, 2014.

Hyman, Mark. *The Blood Sugar Solution: The UltraHealthy Program for Losing Weight, Preventing Disease, and Feeling Great Now!* New York: Little, Brown, and Company, 2012.

Johnson, R. J. "Potential Role of Sugar (Fructose) in the Epidemic of Hypertension, Obesity and the Metabolic Syndrome, Diabetes, Kidney Disease, and Cardiovascular Disease." *American Journal of Clinical Nutrition* 86, no. 4 (October 2007): 899–906. http://ajcn.nutrition.org/content/86/4/899.full.

New Hampshire Department of Health and Human Services—Health Promotion in Motion. "How Much Sugar Do You Eat? You May Be Surprised!" dhhs.nh.gov/dphs/nhp/documents/sugar.pdf.

Patz, Aviva. "Is Sugar Really That Bad for You?" *Health*, November 1, 2012. health.com/health/article/0,,20637702,00.html.

Sinatra, Stephen. "Lower High Blood Pressure by Reducing Sugar Intake." Dr. Sinatra. Last reviewed on March 27, 2014. drsinatra.com/lower-high-blood-pressure-by-reducing-sugar-intake.

Wilson, Sarah. *I Quit Sugar: Your Complete 8-Week Detox Program and Cookbook.* New York: Clarkson Potter, 2013.

Dairy

Brostoff, Jonathan, and Linda Gamlin. *Food Allergies and Food Intolerance: The Complete Guide to Their Identification and Treatment.* Rochester, VT: Healing Arts Press, 2000.

Cook, Michelle Schoffro. "11 Reasons to Stop Eating Dairy." Care2 Healthy Living, February 20, 2012. care2.com/greenliving/11-reasons-to-stop-eating-dairy.html.

Hyman, Mark. "Dairy: 6 Reasons You Should Avoid It At All Costs." *Dr. Mark Hyman* (blog), June 24, 2010. http://drhyman.com/blog/2010/06/24/dairy-6-reasons-you-should-avoid-it-at-all-costs-2/.

Sicherer, Scott H. *Food Allergies: A Complete Guide for Eating When Your Life Depends on It.* Baltimore, MD: The Johns Hopkins University Press, 2013.

Dairy and Osteoporosis

"Got Osteoporosis from Milk?" Milk Information Web site. http://milk.elehost.com/html/osteoporosis.html.

Robbins, John. "The Truth about Calcium and Osteoporosis." Food Matters, November 24, 2009. http://foodmatters.tv/articles-1/the-truth-about-calcium-and-osteoporosis.

Yoffe, Emily. "Got Osteoporosis? Maybe All That Milk You've Been Drinking Is to Blame." Slate, August 3, 1999. slate.com/articles/briefing/articles/1999/08/got_osteoporosis.html.

Dairy and Cancer

Cancer Research UK. "Does Milk Cause Cancer?" cancerresearchuk.org/about-cancer/cancers-in-general/cancer-questions/does-milk-cause-cancer.

Chagas, C. E., M. M. Rogero, and L. A. Martini. "Evaluating the Links between Intake of Milk/Dairy Products and Cancer. *Nutrition Reviews* 70, no. 5 (May 2012): 294–300. ncbi.nlm.nih.gov/pubmed/22537215.

Physician's Committee for Responsible Medicine, Food for Life: Cancer Project. "Ask the Expert: Dairy Products." http://pcrm.org/health/cancer-resources/ask/ask-the-expert-dairy-products.

"Recombinant Bovine Growth Hormone." American Cancer Society. Last reviewed on February 18, 2011. cancer.org/cancer/cancercauses/othercarcinogens/athome/recombinant-bovine-growth-hormone.

Caffeine

"Caffeine-Related Health Problems." Thornton Natural Healthcare Centre. Excerpted from *Caffeine Blues: Wake Up to the Hidden Dangers of America's #1 Drug* by Stephen Cherniske. thornton-health.com/articles/caffeine.shtml.

Carpenter, Murray. *Caffeinated: How Our Daily Habit Helps, Hurts, and Hooks Us.* New York: Hudson Street Press, 2014.

Cherniske, Stephen. *Caffeine Blues: Wake Up to the Hidden Dangers of America's #1 Drug.* New York: Warner Books, 1998.

Kovacs, Betty, and Melissa Conrad Stoppler, ed. "Caffeine." MedicineNet.com. Reviewed on December 10, 2013. medicinenet.com/caffeine/article.htm.

Mayo Clinic Staff. "Nutrition and Healthy Eating." Mayo Clinic, April 14, 2014. mayoclinic.org/healthy-living/nutrition-and-healthy-eating/in-depth/caffeine/art-20045678?p=1.

Robbins, Sam. "Top 10 Caffeine-Related Health Problems." HFL Solutions. hflsolutions.com/ne/free_articles/CaffeineProblems_Top10.pdf.

VascularDoc.com. "Vasospasm." vasculardoc.com/vasospasm.aspx.

Wilson, R. E. et al. "A Case of Caffeine-Induced Coronary Artery Vasospasm of a 17-Year-Old Male." Cardiovascular Toxicology 12, no. 2 (June 2012): 175–9. ncbi.nlm.nih.gov/pubmed/22231478.

Alcohol

BioMed Central. "Alcohol Impairs the Body's Ability to Fight Off Viral Infection, Study Finds." ScienceDaily, October 2, 2011. sciencedaily.com/releases/2011/09/110929235156.htm.

Dasgupta, Amitava. *The Science of Drinking: How Alcohol Affects Your Body and Mind.* Lanham, MD: Rowman & Littlefield Publishers, 2011.

"Health Risks of Alcohol: 12 Health Problems Associated with Chronic Heavy Drinking." WebMD. Reviewed on September 15, 2011. webmd.com/mental-health/addiction/features/12-health-risks-of-chronic-heavy-drinking?page=2.

Kuhn, Cynthia, Scott Swartzwelder, and Wilkie Wilson. *Buzzed: The Straight Facts about the Most Used and Abused Drugs from Alcohol to Ecstasy.* 4th ed. New York: W.W. Norton & Company, 2014.

National Institute on Alcohol Abuse and Alcoholism. "Alcohol's Effects on the Body." niaaa.nih.gov/alcohol-health/alcohols-effects-body.

National Institute on Alcohol Abuse and Alcoholism. *Beyond Hangovers: Understanding Alcohol's Impact on Your Health.* NIH Publication No 13-7604, September 2010. http://pubs.niaaa.nih.gov/publications/Hangovers/beyondHangovers.htm.

Szabo, G. "Consequences of Alcohol and Consumption on Host Defence." *Alcohol and Alcoholism* 34, no. 6 (1999): 830–41. http://alcalc.oxfordjournals.org/content/34/6/830.full.

World Health Organization. "Harmful Use of Alcohol." NMH Fact Sheet, June 2009. who.int/nmh/publications/fact_sheet_alcohol_en.pdf.

Chapter 5 Cleaning from the Inside Out

Baillie-Hamilton, P. F. "Chemical Toxins: A Hypothesis to Explain the Global Obesity Epidemic." *Journal of Alternative and Complementary Medicine* 8, no. 2 (April 2002): 185–92. ncbi.nlm.nih.gov/pubmed/12006126.

Baker, Anne. "Ten Signals Your Liver Is Telling You You Need to Detox." *Nourish Holistic Nutrition* (blog), November 29, 2012. http://nourishholisticnutrition.com/ten-signals-your-liver-is-telling-you-you-need-to-detox/.

Bruno, Gene. "Detoxification: Dietary Supplements to Support & Promote the Process— Informed Opinion." Natural Health Research Institute, 2014. naturalhealthresearch.org/detoxification-dietary-supplements-to-support-promote-the-process/.

Carahealth—Online Naturopathic Health Resource. "Phase 1 and 2 Liver Detoxification Pathways." carahealth.com/health-conditions-a-to-z/digestive-system/detox/365-phase-1-and-2-liver-detoxification-pathways60.html.

Colborn, T., F. S. vom Saal, and A. M. Soto. "Developmental Effects of Endocrine-Disrupting Chemicals in Wildlife and Humans. *Environmental Health Perspectives* 101, no. 5 (October 1993): 378–84. ncbi.nlm.nih.gov/pmc/articles/PMC1519860/pdf/envhper00375-0020.pdf.

Finn, Alison. "Cleansing the Organs of Elimination." Living Foods. livingfoods.co.uk/pages/articles/inner-cleansing.php.

Gelula, Melisse. "5 Signs You Might Need a Detox This Fall." Well+Good, August 30, 2013. wellandgoodnyc.com/2013/08/5-signs-you-might-need-a-detox-this-fall/.

Grandjean, P., and P. Landrigan. "Neurobehavioural Effects of Developmental Toxicity." *The Lancet Neurology* 13, no. 3 (March 2014): 330–38. doi:10.1016/S1474-4422(13)70278-3.

Group, Edward F. "14 Foods That Cleanse the Liver." Global Healing Center, updated May 5, 2014. globalhealingcenter.com/natural-health/liver-cleanse-foods/.

Group, Edward F. "Symptoms of Liver Toxicity." Global Healing Center, updated February 13, 2014. globalhealingcenter.com/natural-health/symptoms-of-liver-toxicity/.

Healthline Editorial Team. "Body Maps: Liver." Healthline. Reviewed on April 24, 2013. healthline.com/human-body-maps/liver.

Hepatitis B Foundation. "Your Liver and How It Works." hepb.org/pdf/the_liver.pdf.

"Is Your House Making You Sick?" WebMD, 2003. webmd.com/women/features/reduce-toxins-in-your-home.

Jade, Kathleen. "Liver Detox: Why You Need It . . . How to Do It." *Mother Earth News Natural Health* (blog), August 5, 2013. motherearthnews.com/natural-health/liver-detox-zbcz1308.aspx.

Life Extension Foundation for Longer Life. "Metabolic Detoxification: Additional Aspects of the Detoxification Process." lef.org/protocols/metabolic_health/metabolic_detoxification_02.htm.

Loecher, Barbara. "Scary Stuff in Your Home." *Prevention*, December 2011. prevention.com/health/healthy-living/protect-yourself-toxins-your-home.

Merrell, Woodson, with Mary Beth Augustine and Hillari Dowdle. *The Detox Prescription: Supercharge Your Health, Strip Away Pounds, and Eliminate the Toxins Within*. New York: Rodale, 2013.

Mitchell, Traci D. "10 Foods That Detox Your Body and Cleanse Your Liver." Get Fit Chicago, December 10, 2013. chicagonow.com/get-fit-chicago/2013/12/10-foods-that-detox-your-body-and-cleanse-your-liver/.

NDHealthFacts. "Elimination of Toxins." Updated February 19, 2014. ndhealthfacts.org/wiki/Elimination_of_Toxins.

Newbold, Retha R., Elizabeth Padilla-Banks, Wendy N. Jefferrson, and Jerrold J. Heindel. "Effects of Endocrine Disruptors on Obesity." *International Journal of Andrology* 31, no. 2 (April 2008): 201–8. ncbi.nlm.nih.gov/pubmed/18315718.

Ortho Molecular pamphlet. "Core Restore Patient Guide: Revitalizing Healthy Liver Function," Woodstock, Illinois.

Park, Alice. "Top 10 Common Household Toxins: The Hazards Lurking at Home." *Time*, April 1, 2010. http://content.time.com/time/specials/packages/article/0,28804,1976909_1976895_1976914,00.html.

Patel, Arti. "Foods for Liver: 20 Detoxing Things to Cook with This Year." *Huffington Post Canada*, updated January 25, 2014. huffingtonpost.ca/2013/12/31/foods-for-liver-_n_4524277.html.

Summerly, John. "36 Foods That Help Detox and Cleanse Your Entire Body." One Radio Network, January 1, 2014. http://oneradionetwork.com/latest/36-foods-that-help-detox-and-cleanse-your-entire-body-3-article/.

"Toxins and the Liver." The Borneo Post, http://netinc.net.my/health/l/002.htm.

US Department of Health and Human Services. *The Surgeon General's Call to Action to Prevent and Decrease Overweight and Obesity*. Rockville, MD: DHHS, Public Health Service, Office of the Surgeon General, 2001. ncbi.nlm.nih.gov/books/NBK44206/.

Wolfe, David. *Eating for Beauty*. Berkeley, CA: North Atlantic Books, 2009.

Chapter 7 The 14-Day Liver Cleanse

Academy of Nutrition and Dietetics. "Aztec Diet Secret: What Are Chia Seeds?" Reviewed on April 2013. eatright.org/Public/content.aspx?id=6442472548.

Food Matters. "16 Health Benefits of Drinking Warm Lemon Water." January 2, 2014. http://foodmatters.tv/articles-1/cheers-to-drinking-warm-lemon-water.

Hathwell, Jen. "Top 10 Health Benefits of Chia Seeds." *SFGate*. http://healthyeating. sfgate.com/top-10-health-benefits-chia-seeds-6962.html.

"19 Ways to Measure Perfect and Healthy Portion Sizes." *Women's Health*. womenshealthmag. com/printwhlist?nid=37301.

Sampath, Pavitra. "10 Reasons to Drink Warm Water with Lemon and Honey in the Morning." The Health Site, February 6, 2014. thehealthsite.com/diseases-conditions/why-drinking-water-early-in-the-morning-good-for-health-p214/.

Zelman, Kathleen. "WebMD Portion-Size Guide." Reviewed on September 27, 2012. webmd.com/diet/printable/wallet-portion-control-size-guide.

Chapter 8 The Clean Up Your Act Diet

American Heart Association. "Understanding Food Nutrition Labels." Last reviewed in October 2014. heart.org/HEARTORG/GettingHealthy/NutritionCenter/ HeartSmartShopping/Reading-Food-Nutrition-Labels_UCM_300132_Article.jsp.

Body Ecology. "Mercury in Your Diet May Cause Fatty Liver Disease." September 20, 2011. http://bodyecology.com/articles/mercury-in-your-diet.

Borrell, Brendan. "Bisphenol A Link to Heart Disease Confirmed: Second Study Supports an Association between the Chemical and Cardiovascular Problems." *Nature*, published online January 13, 2010. nature.com/news/2010/100113/full/ news.2010.7.html.

Boyles, Salynn. "Study: High BPA Linked to Sex Problems in Men: Men Exposed to High Levels of the Chemical Reported Erection Problems, Lower Sex Drive." WebMD, 2009. webmd.com/erectile-dysfunction/news/20091111/study-high-bpa-linked-to-sex-issues-in-men.

Breast Cancer Fund. "Parabens." breastcancerfund.org/clear-science/radiation-chemicals-and-breast-cancer/parabens.html.

Burwell, Sylvia. "13th Report on Carcinogens (RoC)." US Department of Health and Human Services National Toxicology Program, October 2, 2014. http://ntp.niehs. nih.gov/ntp/roc/twelfth/profiles/butylatedhydroxyanisole.pdf.

Calton, Jayson, and Mira Calton. "8 Additives from the US That Are Banned in Other Countries." Food Matters, June 24, 2013. http://foodmatters.tv/articles-1/8-additives-from-the-us-that-are-banned-in-other-countries.

Darbre, P. D. "Concentrations of Parabens in Human Breast Tumours." *Journal of Applied Toxicology* 24, no. 1 (January–February 2004): 5–13. ncbi.nlm.nih.gov/ pubmed/14745841.

Doherty, L. et al. "In Utero Exposure to Diethylstilbestrol (DES) or Bisphenol-A (BPA) Increases EZH2 Expression in the Mammary Gland: An Epigenetic Mechanism Linking Endocrine Disruptors to Breast Cancer." *Hormones and Cancer* 1, no. 3 (June 2010): 146–55. ncbi.nlm.nih.gov/pmc/articles/PMC3140020/.

EPA. "How People Are Exposed to Mercury." Last updated on March 10, 2014. epa.gov/ mercury/exposure.htm.

"EWG's 2014 Shopper's Guide to Pesticides in Produce." Environmental Working Group, April 2014. ewg.org/foodnews/list.php.

Hocman, G. Chemoprevention of Cancer: Phenolic Antioxidants (BHT, BHA)." *International Journal of Biochemistry* 20, no. 7 (1988): 639–51. ncbi.nlm.nih.gov/pubmed/3053283.

Li, D. et al. "Occupational Exposure to Bisphenol-A (BPA) and the Risk of Self-Reported Male Sexual Dysfunction." *Human Reproduction* 25, no. 2 (February 2010): 519–27. Complete article at oxfordjournals.org/news/dep381.pdf?origin=publicationDetail.

Natural Resources Defense Council. "Bush Mercury Policy Threatens the Health of Women and Children." Press release, February 27, 2004. nrdc.org/media/pressreleases/040227.asp.

Natural Resources Defense Council. "Mercury Contamination in Fish: A Guide to Staying Healthy and Fighting Back; Consumer Guide to Mercury in Fish." nrdc.org/health/effects/mercury/guide.asp.

Natural Resources Defense Council. "Mercury Contamination in Fish: A Guide to Staying Healthy and Fighting Back; Learn About Mercury and Its Effects." nrdc.org/health/effects/mercury/effects.asp.

Rabin, Roni Caryn. "Sorting Out the Risks of Fish." *The Consumer* (blog), *New York Times*, March 17, 2014. http://well.blogs.nytimes.com/2014/03/17/sorting-out-the-risks-of-fish/?_php=true&_type=blogs&_r=0.

Soto, A. M., and C. Sonnenschein. "Environmental Causes of Cancer: Endocrine Disruptors as Carcinogens." *Nature Reviews Endocrinology* 6 (July 2010): 363–70. nature.com/nrendo/journal/v6/n7/full/nrendo.2010.87.html.

"Top Dirty Dozen and Clean 15 Foods." *Huffington Post*, April 30, 2014. huffingtonpost.ca/2014/04/30/top-dirty-dozen-and-clean_n_5242343.html.

Zerbe, Leah. "BPA Now, Heart Disease Later." *Prevention*, February 2012. prevention.com/health/health-concerns/bpa-linked-heart-disease-study.

Chapter 9 Any Time, Any Place: Practical Tips to Make It Work

Allrich, Karina. "Gluten-Free Baking Tips + Substitutes." *Gluten-Free Goddess Recipes* (blog). http://glutenfreegoddess.blogspot.com/2008/12/baking-cooking-substitutions-for-gluten.html.

"Food Substitute Guide." Gluten Free Works. http://glutenfreeworks.com/diet-and-health/food-substitutes.

Jaret, Peter. "Reading the Ingredient Label: What to Look For." WebMD. Reviewed on October 20, 2008. webmd.com/food-recipes/features/healthy-ingredients.

Morin, Kate. "27 Gluten-Free Recipe Substitutions." Greatist, December 27, 2011. http://greatist.com/health/27-gluten-free-recipe-substitutions.

Novak, Sara. "7 Dangerous Food Additives and Ingredients and How to Avoid Them." HowStuffWorks. http://blog.xuite.net/greenisfuture/hkblog/115031406-7+Dangerous+Food+Additives+and+Ingredients+and+How+to+Avoid+Them.

Packet to Packet Conversions (adapted for use in this book). CookingWithStevia.com. cookingwithstevia.com/stevia_conversion_chart.html.

Perry, Cat. "The 9 Scariest Food Additives You're Eating Right Now." *Men's Fitness*, March 27, 2014. mensfitness.com/nutrition/avoid-these-9-worst-food-ingredients.

Shakeshaft, Jordan. "30 Dairy-Free Recipe Substitutions." Greatist, December 15, 2011. http://greatist.com/health/30-dairy-free-recipe-substitutions.

US Food and Drug Administration. "How to Understand and Use the Nutrition Facts Label." Updated June 18, 2014. fda.gov/Food/IngredientsPackagingLabeling/LabelingNutrition/ucm274593.htm.

Zinczenko, David, with Matt Goulding. "Eight Ingredients You Never Want to See on Your Nutrition Label." *Men's Health*, August 23, 2012. http://wakeup-world.com/2012/10/05/eight-ingredients-you-never-want-to-see-on-your-nutrition-label/.

Chapter 10 No-Fuss Recipes

I read these cookbooks and Web sites for inspiration:

Credicott, Tammy. *The Healthy Gluten-Free Life: 200 Delicious Gluten-Free, Dairy-Free, Soy-Free & Egg-Free Recipes*. Las Vegas: Victory Belt Publishers, 2012.

Ferreira, Charity. *Perfect Pops*. San Francisco, CA: Chronicle Books, 2011.

Guest, Cornelia. *Cornelia Guest's Simple Pleasures: Healthy Seasonal Cooking & Easy Entertaining*. New York: Weinstein Books, 2012.

Heller, Ricki. *Naturally Sweet & Gluten-Free: Allergy-Friendly Vegan Desserts*. South Portland, ME: Sellers Publishing, Inc., 2013.

Hunn, Nicole. *Gluten-Free on a Shoestring: 125 Easy Recipes for Eating Well on the Cheap*. New York: Da Capo Press, 2011.

Jones, Marjorie Hurt. *The Allergy Self-Help Cookbook: Over 350 Natural Food Recipes, Free of All Common Food Allergens*. Rev. ed. New York: Rodale, 2001.

O'Brien, Susan. *Gluten-Free, Sugar-Free Cooking: Over 200 Delicious Recipes to Help You Live a Healthier, Allergy-Free Life*. New York: Marlow & Company, 2006.

http://epicurious.com/recipesmenus

http://food.com/recipes

http://marthastewart.com/food

http://oprah.com/food

http://taste.com.au/kitchen/recipes

http://tasteofhome.com/recipes

Well (blog), *New York Times*, http://well.blogs.nytimes.com

INDEX

Underscored page references indicate sidebars. **Boldface** references indicate illustrations.